GLUTEN FREE ANYTIME

First Edition - March, 1989
Second Printing - February 1991
Third Printing - July 1993
Fourth Revision & Reprinting - October, 1995
Fifth Revision & Reprinting - July 1997

ISBN O-9694581-1-8

*These Celiac Recipes
have been
written and tested
by
Joyce Friesen
B.Ed., H.Ec.*

*The Cookbook
has been
typed and published
by
Donna Wall
R.N.*

Revised edition of Gluten Free Anytime is dedicated to the memory of Joyce Friesen who dedicated many hours in the development of these recipes.

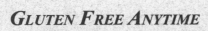 

GLUTEN FREE ANYTIME

TABLE OF CONTENTS

GLUTEN FREE ANYTIME

QUICK BREADS

Muffins

Biscuits

Loaves

GLUTEN FREE ANYTIME

GLUTEN FREE ANYTIME

SQUARES

GLUTEN FREE ANYTIME

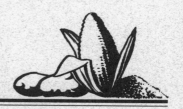

GLUTEN FREE ANYTIME

PASTRY AND PIES

DESSERTS

GLUTEN FREE ANYTIME

MAIN DISHES

GLUTEN FREE ANYTIME

FOREWORD

"Gluten Free Anytime" is a cookbook dedicated to those individuals who have developed an intolerance to gluten. Gluten is found in products derived from wheat, oats, rye, and barley. This condition is called Celiac Disease. The treatment .... a gluten free diet for life.

As the artistic theme throughout the cookbook we have developed a logo illustrating the typical substitutes for gluten products; corn, potatoes, and rice.

There is considerable difficulty in achieving palatable cooked and baked food on a gluten free diet. The objective of "Gluten Free Anytime" is to give those who must be on a gluten- free diet a more varied and tasty selection of basic baked and cooked products. We have attempted to present the recipes in a simple and easy to understand format.

This cookbook encompasses food recipes that usually require flour in their preparation like loaves, cakes, and breads. We feel Celiacs will enjoy these new foods and food ideas. Recipes for salads, vegetables, and most main courses can be found in regular cookbooks.

PLEASE NOTE: Severe medical problems to Celiacs may occur if any ingredient used includes gluten. It is up to the individual to ensure that all products and ingredients are gluten free.

METRIC CONVERSIONS

Standard Metric Conversions for Baking and Cooking (not exact conversions)

<u>Measurements (ml is milliliter)</u>

1/4 tsp	1 ml
1/2 tsp	2 ml
3/4 tsp	3 ml
1 tsp	5 ml
1 tbsp	15 ml
1/4 cup	50 ml
1/3 cup	75 ml
1/2 cup	125 ml
2/3 cup	150 ml
3/4 cup	175 ml
1 cup	250 ml
1 1/2 cup	375 ml
2 cup	500 ml
1 oz	30 grams
3 oz	85 grams
8 oz	250 grams
16 oz	500 grams

GLUTEN FREE ANYTIME

Bakeware

8 x 8	20 x 20 cm
9 x 9	22 x 22 cm
9 x 5 x 3 (loaf)	23 x 12 x 7 cm
9 x 13	22 x 33 cm
7 x 11	17 x 28 cm

Oven Temperature

200 F	75 C
275 F	140 C
300 F	150 C
325 F	160 C
350 F	180 C
375 F	190 C
400 F	200 C
425 F	220 C
450 F	230 C

GLUTEN FREE BAKING HINTS

1. Gluten is that portion of flour that holds ingredients together and forms the structure of the baked product. Gluten free flours are lacking this structuring to a great extent.

2. Binders help to improve the structuring. Eggs, gelatin, and gums are used quite successfully.

3. Baking is affected by temperature and altitude. On a hot day or in a hot kitchen, baking with a lot of margarine, butter or shortening will give the dough or batter a more liquid consistency. Pastry is most affected. Cold ingredients are necessary.

4. Measure carefully using level measurements.

5. Remember to sift flours, starches, and mix before measuring and then sift together again. Generally, sifting improves the texture of the product.

6. A combination of flours/starches seem to produce the best product.

7. Bananas, fruits, nuts, applesauce, yogurt, and honey seem to improve a "floury" look.

8. Products using only rice flour are improved by "sitting" in the refrigerator for 1/2 hour before cooking or baking as in crepes.

9. Tapioca starch and potato starch can be interchanged quite successfully.

** Potato starch and potato flour are two very different ingredients when used in baking and cooking. The starch is very white in appearance and is light and airy. Potato flour is creamy white and heavy in texture and absorbs much more liquid.

10. Potato flour (not Casco) is a good thickener for making scalloped dishes. Casco flour is 100% potato starch.

11. Eggs separate best while cool, but should be at room temperature to achieve the best volume when beaten. This is especially true when making angel, chiffon, and sponge cakes.

12. Use a little cocoa when you have to grease and "flour" a pan for baking a chocolate cake. This avoids a "floury" look.

13. After baking wrap the product when only just cool. Gluten-free baking dries out quickly. Wrap well to store in the refrigerator for only 2 - 4 days; otherwise freeze.

14. Gluten-free products are quite perishable and will mold quickly because the flours and baked products contain no preservatives.

15. When freezing fruit pies, especially berry pies, more thickening needs to be used as starch weakens on freezing. Use double the amount of thickening for juicy fruit pies. Do not cut vents in top of pie crust until ready to bake.

16. Mix cornstarch with cold liquid when using it to thicken gravies and sauces.

17. For variety use 1/4 cup ground puffed rice cereal for 1/4 cup rice or soya flour.

** Contact your local Celiac Chapters for information on finding sources of different gluten free flours, and other products used in baking (eg. xanthan gum, sweet rice flour, corn germ)

GLUTEN FREE ANYTIME

GLUTEN- FREE BAKING POWDER

2 parts cream of tartar
1 part baking soda
2 parts cornstarch

Sift all ingredients together so that the mixture is well
blended. Store in an airtight container.

GLUTEN- FREE ICING SUGAR

1 cup granulated sugar
1 tsp cornstarch

With a blender process until the sugar has been ground to a
fine powder. Store in an airtight container.

try ## "GLUTEN FREE ANYTIME" BAKING MIX

3 cups white rice flour
1 cup brown rice flour
2 cups potato starch
1 cup cornstarch
1 cup soya flour

Sift and then measure each amount of flour and starch.
Combine well and store in an airtight container in a cool,
dry place.

Use for cinammon buns too.

BROWN AND WHITE RICE FLOUR BREAD

1 tsp sugar
1/4 cup warm water
1 tbsp (envelope) yeast

Dissolve sugar in warm water. Sprinkle yeast over water. Stir briefly. Let sit for 10 minutes until foamy on top.

1 1/2 cups brown rice flour
1 1/2 cups white rice flour
1 tsp salt
1 tbsp xanthan gum
2/3 cup dry milk powder

Mix these dry ingredients together in a large bowl.

1 1/4 cup warm water
1/4 cup margarine

Melt margarine in the warm water. Add this mixture to the softened yeast and in turn add this to the dry ingredients. Beat well. Add 3 eggs and beat well for 2 minutes. Cover. Let rise until double (1 - 1 1/2 hours). Beat again for 3 minutes. Pour into 8 1/2 x 4 1/2 greased loaf pan. Let rise until dough reaches the top of pan. Bake at 400 F for 15 minutes, cover with foil if top is getting too brown. Continue baking for about 45 minutes longer. Remove from pan and leave unwrapped just until cool.

GLUTEN FREE ANYTIME

FOR A QUICK BUN

Prepare muffin tins or a 9 x 3 inch pan as above. Shape into buns, let rise and bake at 350 F for about 25 minutes or until slightly browned.

RAISIN BREAD

1/2 cup raisins
1 1/2 tsp cinnamon
1/4 cup sugar

Add above to original dry ingredients. Then bake as for above recipe.

GLUTEN FREE BREAD

1 tsp sugar
1 tbsp (envelope) traditional yeast
1/4 cup warm water

Dissolve sugar in warm water. Sprinkle yeast over the water. Let sit covered for 10 minutes until foamy on top.

1 cup white rice flour
1 cup brown rice flour
1 cup potato starch
1/2 cup instant mashed potato
2/3 cup dry milk powder
1 tsp salt
2 tbsp psyllium hydrophilic mucilloid
(Metamucil)

Mix these dry ingredients together in large mixing bowl.

1 1/4 cup warm water (or potato water if you have any)
1/4 cup margarine
3 eggs

Melt margarine in the warm water. Add this water margarine mixture to the softened yeast and in turn add this to the dry ingredients. Beat well. Add eggs and beat for about 2 minutes. Scrape down the dough from the sides of the bowl. Cover bowl with buttered saran wrap. Place in an oven which has been heated to 200 F and then turned off. Let rise until double (about 1-1 1/2 hours). Beat dough again for about 2 - 3 minutes. Place in a greased 8 1/2 x 4 1/2 inch loaf pan. Let rise again until dough reaches the top of pan. Preheat oven to 375 F. Bake for 1 hour. Let sit for 5 minutes on rack, remove from pan and leave unwrapped just until cool.

CINNAMON ROLLS

The dough is made using the Brown and White Rice Flour Bread recipe.

The dough is stiff enough that it can be patted flat and rolled up like a cinnamon roll and cut. While dough is rising spread the following mixture into a greased 9 x 13 inch pan:

1/4 to 1/2 cup melted margarine or butter
1/2 cup brown sugar
1 - 2 tbsp water to dissolve brown sugar
1/2 cup raisins

When the dough has risen punch dough down with wet hands. Lay the dough on a board or cupboard which has been greased with melted butter or margarine. Pat dough to a 12 x 14 inch rectangle with wet hands. Spread 1/4 cup melted butter over dough, and cover with a mixture of 1 1/2 tsp cinnamon and 1/2 cup brown sugar. Gently roll dough up into log with damp hands, cut into 1 inch slices with a sharp knife dipped in cool water. Place slices into the prepared pan. Let rise 1/2 hour and bake at 350 until slightly browned about 25 - 30 minutes. Makes 12 - 14 rolls.

CINNAMON PECAN NUT ROLLS

To the dry ingredients of the brown and white bread recipe add:

1/3 - 1/2 cup brown sugar
1 tsp cinnamon
2 tbsp xanthan gum instead of 1 tbsp
1/2 cup raisins

Follow instructions for brown and white bread; prepare muffin tins while dough is rising. In bottom of each tin put the following ingredients:

1 tbsp melted margarine
2 tbsp brown sugar
1 tbsp chopped walnuts or pecans
1/4 tsp cinnamon

After letting rise, shape into buns and let rise for 1/2 hour again. Bake at 350 F for 25-30 minutes.

MICROWAVE METHOD OF RISING BREAD

Put the bread mixture into a greased glass (pyrex) bowl. Seal well with saran wrap. Put over a glass pie pan which is filled with lukewarm water and place in the microwave at the lowest setting for 30 minutes. Remove from microwave, beat mixture 3 minutes as stated in the recipe, pour into the prepared pans. Return to the microwave oven but do not turn any power on and let the bread rise until the dough reaches the top of pans. (pans can be the usual metal)

GLUTEN FREE ANYTIME

TRAVEL BREAD MIX

1 cup brown rice flour
2 cups white rice flour
1/4 cup sugar
1 tbsp xanthan gum
2/3 cup dry milk powder
1 1/2 tsp salt
1 tbsp (envelope) fast (quick) rise yeast

Combine the above ingredients. When ready to make bread add 1 3/4 cups warm water, 1/4 cup margarine melted, in the water and then 2 eggs. Beat well for 2 minutes. Let rise until double (1 - 1 1/2 hours). Beat again for 3 minutes. Pour dough into 2 greased small or 1 large pan. Let rise until dough is slightly above top of pan. Bake at 400 F for 10 minutes. Place foil over bread and bake 50 minutes more. Remove from pan and leave unwrapped just until cool.

BREAD MACHINE

WHITE BAKERY BREAD

2 eggs, beaten
1 1/2 cups tap water
1 tsp lemon juice or vinegar (preservative)
1/4 cup oil (can use 2 tbsp if on low fat diet)
1 1/2 cups white rice flour
1 cup brown rice flour
1/2 cup tapioca starch
2 tsp granulated sugar
1 tsp salt
2 tsp xanthan gum
1/2 cup milk powder
1 tbsp fast rising yeast

Sift and mix dry ingredients together in a bowl. Add wet ingredients. Beat by hand until mixed. Pour into bread machine baking canister. Bake on either 3 or 4 hour cycle. Let cool completely before removing loaf from canister.

Variations:
Cheese Bread - add 1/2 cup coarsely grated sharp cheese
Cinnamon Bread - add 1/2 cup raisins and 1 tsp cinnamon
Sesame Bread - add 3 tbsp toasted sesame seeds or 3 tbsp sunflower seeds

** Bread baker recipes tested in Panasonic and Hitachi bread bakery machines.**

BREAD MACHINE

very nice

BROWN BAKERY BREAD

2 eggs
1 cup water
3/4 cup milk
1/4 cup oil
1 tbsp molasses
3/4 cup white rice flour
3/4 cup brown rice flour
3/4 cup potato starch
2 tsp white sugar
1 tbsp brown sugar
1 tbsp xanthan gum
1 tsp salt
1/4 cup rolled rice or 1/4 cup rice bran
1 tbsp fast rising yeast

Aileen - Mix seperately in bowls not in bread machine. set at Whole Wheat Rapid

Sift and mix dry ingredients together in a bowl. Add wet ingredients. Beat by hand until mixed. Pour into bread machine baking canister. Bake on either 3 or 4 hour cycle. Let cool completely before removing loaf from canister.
Variations:
Buckwheat Bread - substitute 1/4 cup buckwheat for rolled rice
Substitute 1 tbsp Roger's Golden syrup for molasses

** Bread baker recipes tested in Panasonic and Hitachi bread bakery machines.**

BREAD MACHINE

DONNA'S IMPROVED RICE BREAD

1 1/4 cups cold water
1 tbsp cold margarine or butter
2 eggs
1/4 cup sour cream

1/4 cup cornstarch
1/2 cup potato starch
1 cup rice flour (may use 1/2 white and 1/2 brown)
1 tsp salt
1/2 cup skim milk powder
1/2 tbsp xanthan gum
1 tsp sugar
1 1/2 tsp fast rising yeast

Sift and mix dry ingredients together in bowl. Add wet ingredients. Beat by hand until mixed. Pour into bread machine baking canister. Bake on 4 hour cycle. Let cool completely before removing loaf from canister. Makes 1 small loaf. Tastes great warm with butter!

Bread baker recipes tested in Panasonic and Hitachi bread bakery machines

BASIC MUFFINS

1 1/2 cups "Gluten Free Anytime" Mix
3 tsp baking powder
3/4 tsp salt
2 tbsp sugar

2 eggs, beaten
1/3 cup milk
3 tbsp melted margarine

Preheat oven to 425 F. Sift baking mix and measure. Sift all dry ingredients into a medium sized mixing bowl. Mix milk, margarine, and eggs together, and stir in just until blended. Spoon into greased muffin tins 2/3 full. Bake for 15 - 20 minutes.

Variations -

1/2 cup raisins, 1/2 cup coarsely grated cheese, 1/2 cup chopped nuts, or blueberries may be added to the dry ingredients of the above basic recipe to give you a variety of muffins.

BLUEBERRY MUFFINS

good

1 cup white rice flour
1/2 cup potato starch
3 tsp baking powder
1/4 tsp salt
1/2 cup sugar (granulated)

1 egg
1 egg yolk
1/2 cup milk
1/3 cup melted margarine
1 tbsp lemon rind, grated
1 cup blueberries, fresh or frozen

Preheat oven to 400 F. Grease 12 medium muffin tins. In a mixing bowl sift and mix together flours, salt, sugar, and baking powder. In a smaller bowl, beat egg, egg yolk, then add milk and melted margarine. Add liquids to dry ingredients all at once; stir just until moistened. Stir in blueberries and grated lemon rind. Spoon into prepared muffin tins to 3/4 full. Bake at 400 F for about 20 minutes. Makes 12 medium muffins.

CHEESY APPLESAUCE MUFFINS

2 cups brown rice flour
1/4 cup corn germ
2 tbsp sugar
4 tsp baking powder
1/2 tsp baking soda
1/4 tsp salt

1/4 cup soft margarine
2 eggs, slightly beaten
3/4 cup milk
3/4 cup applesauce
1 1/2 cups grated cheddar cheese

Preheat oven to 400 F. Combine dry ingredients together. Cut in margarine until mixture is crumbly. Add grated cheese.

Combine liquid ingredients together. Pour all at once over dry ingredients.Stir quickly until just blended. Batter will be lumpy. Fill greased muffin tins 3/4 full. Bake at 400 for 18 -20 minutes. Makes 12 large muffins.

LIGHT APPLE BRAN MUFFINS

1/4 cup margarine
3/8 cup sugar
2 tbsp molasses
2 eggs

1 1/4 cups brown rice flour
1/4 cup rice bran
2 tsp baking powder
1/2 tsp baking soda
pinch salt
1/2 cup buttermilk
1 small apple, peeled & chopped

Preheat oven to 425 F. Cream margarine and sugar. Add molasses, then eggs and beat well. Add chopped apple. Sift dry ingredients and add alternately with buttermilk. Stir just until mixed. Bake for approximately 15 - 18 minutes in greased muffin tins. Makes 16 muffins.

Alternative ideas -

1. Add apple or blueberry pie filling instead of apple.
2. Can use very ripe banana.

BANANA BRAN MUFFINS

1 egg, beaten
1/3 cup oil
1/4 cup buttermilk
1/4 cup brown sugar
1 cup mashed bananas

3/4 cup soya flour
3/4 cup brown rice flour
1/4 cup rice bran
1 tsp baking soda
3 tsp baking powder
1 tsp unflavored gelatin
1/4 tsp nutmeg
1/2 cup chopped nuts (opt)

Preheat oven to 425 F. Sift dry ingredients together in
mixing bowl. Mix beaten egg, oil, and bananas together.
Add all at once to dry ingredients. Stir just until blended -
add nuts if desired. Bake in greased muffin tins 3/4 full for
15 - 20 minutes. Makes 10 - 12 muffins.

BANANA MUFFINS

1/2 cup margarine or butter
1/2 cup white sugar
1/4 cup brown sugar
2 eggs, beaten
1 tsp vanilla

1 tsp baking soda
4 tbsp sour cream
1 cup mashed banana
1/4 tsp salt
1 1/2 cups "Gluten Free Anytime" Baking Mix
1/2 cup chocolate chips or 1/2 cup chopped walnuts (opt)

Cream butter, sugar, vanilla, and then add the eggs. Mix the baking soda and sour cream together and refrigerate for 1 hour. Add the chilled baking soda mixture to the butter-sugar mixture and beat well. (If using chocolate chips or walnuts add them to the dry ingredients). Add the bananas, flour, and salt. Mix well, then pour batter into greased muffin tins 3/4 full. Bake at 400 F for 15 - 20 minutes. Makes 18 muffins.

SPICY PUMPKIN MUFFINS

1 1/2 cups brown rice flour
3 tsp baking powder
1/2 cup potato starch
1 tsp unflavored gelatin
1 tsp ginger
1 tsp cinnamon
1/2 tsp salt

Sift above ingredients together. Then beat together:

1/4 cup honey
1/2 cup melted margarine
2 eggs
1/2 cup fruit juice
1/2 cup pumpkin (cooked)

Preheat oven to 375 F.
Add liquids to dry ingredients. Mix quickly and spoon into greased muffin tins. Bake at 375 F for 15 - 20 minutes.

SOUR CREAM CHOCOLATE MUFFINS/CAKE

2 eggs
1 cup sugar
1 cup sour cream
1 tsp vanilla

1 tsp baking powder
1/2 cup soya flour
pinch of salt
1 cup rice flour
1/2 cup cocoa
1 tsp baking soda in 1/2 cup hot water

Preheat oven to 350 F. Grease 12 muffin cups.
Beat eggs, adding sugar, and beat well. Mix with dry
ingredients; then add sour cream and vanilla. Mix hot
water with baking soda and add to other ingredients. Mix
with electric mixer for 3 minutes. Fill muffin cups 2/3 full.
Bake at 350 F for 25 - 30 minutes.

try

CARROT MUFFINS

1 egg, beaten
1/2 cup milk
1/3 cup melted margarine
1/4 cup brown sugar

1 cup brown rice flour
1/2 cup cornstarch   *potatoestarch*
2 tsp baking powder
1 tsp baking soda
1 tsp cinnamon
1/4 tsp ginger
1/2 tsp salt

1/2 cup raisins or nuts (opt)
1 1/4 cups grated carrots

Preheat oven to 400 F. Sift dry ingredients together in mixing bowl, except brown sugar. Mix beaten egg, margarine, and sugar together, then add milk. Add all at once to dry ingredients just until blended. Stir in carrots, nuts or raisins last. Bake at 400 for 15 -20 minutes. Makes 12 muffins.

SOUR CREAM MUFFINS

Topping: 1 tbsp sugar and 1 tsp cinnamon

Batter: 2 cups "Gluten Free Anytime" Mix
              1/2 cup sugar
              4 tsp baking powder
              1/2 tsp salt
              1/4 tsp baking soda
              1/2 cup sour cream
              1/4 cup melted margarine
              1/2 cup milk
              1 egg

Preheat oven to 375 F. Grease muffin pans. Mix
together topping ingredients and set aside. Sift dry ingredients into mixing bowl. Set aside. Beat egg until thick, add
remaining ingredients and blend well. Add all at once to
the dry ingredients. Blend well. Spoon batter into prepared
pans, filling 3/4 full. Sprinkle topping on each muffin,
pressing gently into batter with back of spoon. Bake for 18
- 20 minutes. Makes 14-16 muffins.

BREAKFAST MUFFINS

1 cup brown rice flour
1/2 cup tapioca starch
1/2 cup cornflour
1 tsp baking powder
2 tsp baking soda
1/2 tsp salt
1 cup sugar
1/2 tsp unflavored gelatin
2 tsp cinnamon
2 tbsp corn germ
1 apple, peeled and grated
2 cups carrots, peeled and grated
1/2 cup raisins
1/2 cup walnuts, chopped
3 eggs, beaten
3/4 cup vegetable oil
2 tsp vanilla

Preheat oven to 350 F. Grease muffin pans. Combine all dry ingredients which have been sifted together (except for the corn germ). Add grated apple and carrots, raisins, nuts, and corn germ. Beat together eggs, oil and vanilla, and add all at once to the dry ingredients. Stir just to blend all ingredients. Fill muffin cups 3/4 full. Bake for 25 minutes or until top of muffins spring back when lightly touched. Makes 22 muffins.

COFFEE CAKE MUFFINS

1 cup sour cream mixed with 1 tsp baking soda
1/2 cup margarine
3/4 cup sugar
2 eggs
1 tsp vanilla
3/4 cup chocolate chips
1 cup white rice flour
1/2 cup sweet rice flour
1/4 cup potato starch
1/4 cup ground puffed rice
1 1/2 tsp gluten free baking powder
1/4 tsp salt

Topping - mix following ingredients together:
1/4 cup chopped nuts
1/4 cup brown sugar
1/2 tsp cinnamon
2 tsp melted butter

Variations:
Substitute 3/4 cup rhubarb or 3/4 cup frozen blueberries for the chocolate chips for another great taste!

Preheat oven to 375. Sift flours, starch, baking powder and salt together. Set aside. Add baking soda to sour cream and set aside. Cream margarine with sugar, add eggs, vanilla, and beat altogether. Add dry ingredients together with the sour cream mixture, then add chocolate chips. Spoon batter into prepared muffin tins, and top with brown sugar mixture. Bake at 375 F for 20 minutes.

YOGURT TEA BISCUITS

3/4 cup white rice flour
1/2 cup sweet rice flour
1 cup potato starch
3 tsp baking powder
1 tsp baking soda
1/2 tsp salt
5 tbsp butter or margarine
1 - 1 1/8 cup yogurt (can use low fat yogurt)
- use 1 cup first then if necessary add 1/8 cup

Preheat oven to 400 F.   Sift then measure flours and starch
and add along with other dry ingredioents into a bowl (or
food processor) Cut in margarine or butter until the margarine is the size of split peas. Stir in yogurt and blend until
all the dry ingredients are wet. Gather mixture into a ball,
place on a <u>lightly</u> rice floured surface and knead gently
several times. Pat to 1/2 - 3/4 inch thickness. Cut with a
cookie or biscuit cutter. (a glass dipped in rice flour works
well too). Place biscuits on an ungreased baking sheet and
bake 15 minutes approximately.

<u>Variation</u>

1. Add 1/2 cup currants to the mixture when yogurt is
added.

2. Blend 1/4 cup brown sugar (or Sugar Twin Brown sugar substitute) with 1 tsp cinnamon and 1/4 tsp nutmeg. After cutting the biscuits brush with 1 slightly beaten egg and then dip biscuit into brown sugar - spice mixture or sprinkle it on top of each biscuit. Bake at 400 F for about 15 minutes.

TEA BISCUITS

1 1/3 cup white rice flour
2/3 cup potato starch
1 tsp salt
1/2 tsp xanthan gum
1 tsp baking soda
1/2 tsp baking powder
3 tbsp cold butter or marg
1 cup buttermilk

Preheat oven to 400 F.
Sift and mix all dry ingredients. Cut in butter until size of split peas. Add buttermilk. Mix lightly. Pat out to about 3/4 inch thick. Cut out biscuits and place on ungreased baking sheet. Bake for 15-16 minutes.

SODA CRACKERS

1 1/2 cups "Gluten Free Anytime" Mix
1/2 cup sweet rice flour
3/4 tsp xanthan gum
1/2 cup butter
1 tsp salt
1 1/2 tsp vinegar
1/4 tsp baking soda
1/2 cup milk

Preheat oven to 375 F. In a large bowl sift the gluten free mix, sweet rice flour and xanthan gum. Cut in the butter until crumbly. Combine milk, salt, vinegar, and soda. Add slowly to the flour mixture. Mix lightly so the mixture holds together. Roll out very thin. Cut in squares and prick them with a fork. Place on an ungreased baking sheet. Bake for 10 minutes. Toasted sesame seeds may be added to the rolled out dough and then rolled again and pricked with a fork.

CINNAMON ROLLUPS

1 cup soya flour
1 cup brown rice flour
3/4 cup potato starch
1/4 cup sweet rice flour
3 tsp baking powder
1 tsp salt

1/3 cup sugar
1/3 cup butter
1/2 cup evaporated milk
2 eggs, beaten

1/3 cup light brown sugar, packed
1 1/2 tsp cinnamon
1/2 tsp grated orange rind
3 tbsp butter, melted
1/3 cup liquid honey
2/3 cup chopped nuts

Preheat oven to 400 F. Grease muffin tins.
In a large mixing bowl, sift together the flours and starch,
baking powder, salt and sugar. Cut in 1/3 cup butter until
mixture resembles corn meal. Mix evaporated milk and
eggs together.

Add all at once to the dry ingredients, stirring until a soft dough is formed. Turn onto a well rice- floured board and knead 1 minute. To help with rolling, put dough between 2 pieces of saran and roll into a rectangle 10 x 15 inches and about 1/4 inch thick. In a small bowl mix together the brown sugar, cinnamon, orange rind, 3 tbsp melted butter, honey, and chopped pecans. Spread on dough. Roll the dough up tightly jelly roll style with the help of the saran. Cut in one inch slices and arrange each slice, cut side down, in lightly greased muffin cups. Bake in preheated oven at 400 F for 20 minutes. Makes 15 - 20 rolls.

HONEY RICE CRACKERS

1 3/4 cups brown rice flour
(*add 2 tbsp more in a hot kitchen)
1/2 cup sweet rice flour
1 tsp baking powder
3/4 tsp baking soda
1/2 tsp salt
1 tsp xanthan gum

1/2 cup margarine
1/2 cup honey
1 tsp vanilla

Combine flours, baking powder, baking soda, salt and xanthan gum. Set aside. Combine margarine, honey and vanilla in a large bowl and beat until fluffy. Add the dry ingredients to the margarine - honey mixture and blend well. Chill 1 hour.

Preheat oven to 350 F. Roll out crackers on a rice-floured surface, then cut into 2 inch squares. Place on ungreased baking sheets and prick with a fork to resemble graham crackers.

Bake for 10 - 12 minutes. Makes 2 1/2 - 3 dozen.

These crackers can be dried and rolled out to be used instead of graham crumbs as a crust in desserts.

try

BANANA BREAD

1 cup sugar
4 tbsp butter or margarine
2 eggs
1 cup mashed bananas

1 1/2 cups rice flour
1/2 cup cornstarch   OR
Substitute:
1 1/2 cups Gluten Free Anytime Baking Mix
1/2 cup sweet rice flour

1 tsp baking soda
1/4 tsp salt

Preheat oven to 375 F. Grease a 9 x 5 inch loaf pan.

Cream sugar and butter, then add eggs and beat until fluffy.
Sift dry ingredients and add to sugar mixture. Pour into
greased loaf pan. Bake for 50 minutes.

APPLE CHEESE BREAD

1/2 cup margarine
3/8 cup sugar
2 eggs, beaten
2 tbsp yogurt (plain)

1 3/4 cups white rice flour
1/3 cup corn germ
2 tsp baking powder
1/2 tsp baking soda
1/2 tsp salt
1/2 tsp cinnamon
1 tsp unflavored gelatin
1/4 tsp nutmeg
1 1/2 cups apples, peeled and grated
1 1/2 cups sharp cheddar cheese, grated

Preheat oven to 350 F.

Cream margarine, add sugar, eggs and yogurt, then beat until light and fluffy. Blend in apples and cheese. Sift dry ingredients together and add to apple mixture. Mix only until dry ingredients are blended in. Turn into a well greased 8 x 4 x 3 inch loaf pan. Bake for 50 - 60 minutes.

CORN BREAD

1 1/2 cups cornmeal
2 tbsp baking powder
2 cups white rice flour
3/4 tsp salt
1/2 cup sugar

2 eggs, beaten
2 cups milk
1/3 cup melted margarine

Preheat oven to 425 F. Grease 2 - 8 or 9 inch round or square pans.

Sift dry ingredients. Add cornmeal. Beat eggs and add milk and melted margarine. Add liquid ingredients all at once to dry ingredients mixing just to wet dry ingredients. Bake for 20 - 25 minutes.

A piece - 1 1/2 inches is 1 1/2 Starch & 1 Fat exchange.

ZUCCHINI BREAD

2 eggs
1/2 cup oil
1/2 cup sugar
1 cup shredded zucchini

1 1/2 cups brown rice flour
1 tsp cinnamon
1/2 tsp nutmeg
1/4 tsp baking soda
2 tsp baking powder
1 tsp unflavored gelatin
3/4 cup raisins or nuts (optional)

Preheat oven to 350 F. Grease a 9 x 5 loaf pan.

Sift dry ingredients together. Set aside. In a large bowl beat together the eggs, sugar, and oil until light. Add the zucchini. Stir in dry ingredients and nuts or raisins if desired. Bake in a loaf pan at 350 F for approximately 1 hour.

CINNAMON LOAVES

1/2 cup margarine
1 cup sugar
1 tsp vanilla
2 eggs
1 cup dairy sour cream
1/4 cup milk

2 cups "Gluten Free Anytime" Mix
2 1/2 tsp baking powder
1 tsp baking soda
1/2 tsp salt
1 tsp unflavored gelatin

1/2 cup sugar
1 tbsp cinnamon
2 tsp dried orange peel

GLUTEN FREE ANYTIME

Preheat oven to 350 F. Grease 3 - 4 small loaf pans or one large 9 x 5 x 3 inch loaf pan.

In a large mixing bowl cream together the 1 cup sugar and the margarine until light and fluffy. Beat in eggs and vanilla. Add sour cream and milk; beat until mixture is smooth. In mixing bowl stir together the 5 dry ingredients; mix into sour cream mixture till batter is blended. Combine 1/2 cup sugar, cinnamon, and orange peel. Set aside 1/4 of the mixture for topping. Spoon half the batter into prepared loaf pans. Sprinkle the remaining cinnamon mixture over batter; top with remaining batter. With knife cut through batter and cinnamon mixture to swirl. Bake at 350 F for 35 min.for small loaf or 60 min.for large loaf. Cool 10 min in pan, turn onto rack.

PEANUT BUTTER LOAF

2 eggs, beaten
1 cup milk
3/4 cup creamy or chunky peanut butter
1/4 cup melted and cooled margarine

1 cup soya flour
1 cup white rice flour
1/2 cup sugar
3 tsp baking powder
1 tsp salt
1 tsp unflavored gelatin

Preheat oven to 375 F. Grease a 9 x 5 inch loaf pan.

Sift together soya and white rice flour, then sift the flours together with sugar, baking powder, salt and unflavored gelatin into mixing bowl. In another bowl beat the eggs together with melted margarine, peanut butter and milk. Stir liquid ingredients into flour mixture stirring just until dry ingredients are moistened. Pour batter into prepared pan. Bake at 375 F for 1 hour. Cool in pan for 10 minutes; remove from pan and cool on rack covered loosely with a clean towel. (gluten-free baking does not need to be cooled completely before wrapping)

DATE NUT BREAD

1 cup nuts, chopped
1/2 lb dates
1 cup boiling water

2 tbsp margarine or butter
3/4 cup granulated sugar
1 tsp vanilla

1 3/4 cups "Gluten Free Anytime" Mix
1 tsp baking soda
1 tsp cream of tartar
1/2 tsp baking powder
1/2 tsp xanthan gum
pinch salt

Preheat oven to 350 F. Grease 2 small 3 x 6 inch pans or
1 - 9 x 5 inch pan.

Cook nuts, dates, and water together until well blended.
Cool. Sift dry ingredients together, set aside. Cream margarine and sugar well; add vanilla. Add cooled date-nut
mixture to creamed mix. Blend well. Add dry ingredients
and mix until well blended. Bake at 350 F for 45 minutes.

LEMON LOAF

1/2 cup shortening
1 cup granulated sugar
3 eggs
1/4 cup milk
rind of 1 lemon

3/4 cup white rice flour
1/2 cup potato starch
1/4 cup tapioca starch
2 tsp baking powder
1/2 tsp salt

Preheat oven to 350 F. Grease a 9 x 5 inch loaf pan.

Cream shortening, and sugar together well. Add eggs, one
at at time and beat well after each addition. Add lemon
rind, then add sifted dry ingredients alternately with milk.
Pour into prepared pan and bake for 1 hour or until toothpick comes out clean.

Mix lemon juice and 1/2 cup sugar together and glaze loaf
while hot.

APPLESAUCE NUT LOAF

2 eggs, beaten
1/4 cup melted shortening
1 cup unsweetened applesauce
1 cup white rice flour
1/2 cup potato starch
1/2 cup soya flour
3/4 cup sugar
1 tsp unflavored gelatin
1 tsp nutmeg
1/2 tsp cloves
1/2 tsp allspice
3 tsp (1 tbsp) baking powder
1/2 tsp baking soda
1 tsp salt
3/4 cup chopped nuts - walnuts or pecans

Preheat oven to 350 F. Grease a 9 x 5 inch loaf pan.
Sift flours, measure and then sift together with all dry
ingredients. Add nuts. Combine eggs, shortening and
applesauce. Add to the dry ingredients and stir just until
blended. Pour into a loaf pan and bake for 50 - 60 minutes.

APPLESAUCE BREAD (SUGARLESS)

Using the applesauce nut loaf recipe omit the 3/4 cup sugar
and continue with the same format. Serve this bread with
butter or cream cheese.

PUMPKIN SPICE LOAF

3 eggs, beaten
1/3 cup margarine, melted
1/4 cup milk
1 cup sugar
1 cup canned pumpkin

3 tsp baking powder
1 cup white rice flour
1/2 cup cornstarch
1/2 cup soya flour
1 tbsp corn germ
1 tsp baking soda
1 tsp each salt & cinnamon
1/2 tsp nutmeg
1 tsp unflavored gelatin
3/4 cup raisins or 1/2 cup chopped pecans
(optional)

Preheat oven to 350 F. Grease a 9 x 5 inch loaf pan or
2 - 6 x 3 inch loaf pans.

GLUTEN FREE ANYTIME

Sift flours, measure and sift flours together with the remaining dry ingredients except corn germ into a large mixing bowl. Add corn germ and stir to mix. Blend beaten eggs, melted margarine, milk and pumpkin together. Add all at once to the dry ingredients and mix just until blended. (Raisins or nuts are added with the liquids). Spread batter into prepared pan. Bake at 350 F for 1 hour or until toothpick comes out clean when inserted into center or loaf. Cool for 10 minutes on rack, remove from pan. Cool and wrap.

PEANUT BUTTER BREAD (LOAF)

2 eggs
1/2 cup sugar
1/2 cup milk
1/2 cup yogurt

1/2 cup peanut butter
1 cup brown rice flour
1/2 cup potato starch
1/2 cup soya flour
3 tsp baking powder
1/2 tsp salt
1/2 tsp baking soda
1 tsp gelatin (unflavored)

Preheat oven to 350 F. Grease a 9 x 5 inch loaf pan.

Beat eggs until light, add sugar and beat well. Add milk and yogurt. Sift flours, starch, baking powder, salt, baking soda, and gelatin together into a mixing bowl. Add peanut butter to dry ingredients and beat until crumbly. Make a well in center of dry ingredients and add egg mixture. Mix well. Pour into prepared pan and bake for 1 hour. Cool before slicing.

QUICK COFFEE CAKE

1/2 cup milk
1/4 cup melted margarine
1 egg, beaten
1/4 cup sugar

1 cup "Gluten Free Anytime" Mix
3 1/2 tsp baking powder
1/2 tsp salt
1 tsp grated orange rind (opt)

Topping - 2 tbsp sugar and 1 tsp cinnamon, mixed together in a small bowl

Preheat oven to 375 F. Grease well an 8 inch square pan.

Sift, then measure gluten free mix. Sift together mix, sugar, baking powder, and salt into bowl. Stir in grated orange rind if used. Combine beaten egg, milk, and cooled melted margarine in small bowl. Add liquid ingredients all at once to dry ingredients. Stir just until blended and no lumps are visible. Pour into pan. Sprinkle with the cinnamon-sugar mix. Bake at 375 F about 15-20 minutes.

APRICOT STREUSEL COFFEECAKE

1 cup finely chopped dried apricots
1 - 6 oz (1 cup) butterscotch chips
1/2 cup water

1/4 cup brown sugar, packed
1 tbsp white rice flour
1/2 tsp cinnamon
1/2 cup chopped nuts - walnuts or pecans
1 tbsp melted butter

1/4 cup soft margarine
1/2 cup granulated sugar
2 eggs, slightly beaten
1/4 cup milk
1 cup white rice flour
1/2 cup potato starch
3 tsp baking powder
1/2 tsp salt

Combine butterscotch chips, apricots and water. Cook over moderate heat, stirring occcasionally, until thick, about 10 minutes. Cool.

Mix brown sugar, flour (1 tbsp), cinnamon, nuts and melted butter for streusel topping. Set aside.
Preheat oven to 375 F. Grease 9 inch square pan.

Cream soft margarine and sugar together. Add eggs and beat well. Sift together the 1 cup flour, potato starch, baking powder and salt. Add dry ingredients alternately with milk to creamed mixture and mix well. Pour about 2/3 of the batter into prepared pan. Spread cooled apricot mixture over batter. Drop remaining batter in small spoonfuls over filling,. Sprinkle streusel topping over all. Bake 25 minutes. Cool and cut. Serves 8 - 10.

BLUEBERRY COFFEE CAKE

1/2 cup white rice flour
1/4 cup brown rice flour
1/2 cup potato starch
2 tsp baking powder
1/2 cup granulated sugar
1/2 tsp salt

2 eggs, beaten
1/4 cup milk
1/2 tsp vanilla
3 tbsp melted margarine or butter

2 cups fresh or frozen blueberries
1/4 cup brown sugar
1 tsp cinnamon

Preheat oven to 350 F. Grease an 8 x 8 inch square pan.

Mix flours, starch, baking powder, sugar and salt together
and sift into mixing bowl. In a smaller bowl whip eggs, add
milk, vanilla, and melted margarine. Pour into the dry
ingredients and mix thoroughly. Place batter into prepared
pan. Top with blueberries and sprinkle the brown sugar -
cinnamon mixture over the fruit. Bake 35 - 40 minutes.
(Rhubarb may be used in place of blueberries.)

GLUTEN FREE ANYTIME

DOUGHNUTS

3 3/4 cups of "Gluten Free Anytime" Mix
4 tsp baking powder
1/2 tsp salt
1/2 tsp nutmeg
3/4 cup sugar (or 1 cup if you like a sweeter doughnut)
3 tbsp butter or margarine
2 eggs
2/3 cup milk
1 tsp vanilla

Sift flour, then measure and sift flour, baking powder, salt and nutmeg together. Set aside. Cream butter and sugar thoroughly. Add vanilla and blend. Beat in eggs, one at a time. Mix well after each addition. Stir in dry ingredients, alternately with milk, starting and ending with the dry ingredients. Chill dough 1 hour for easier handling. Flour rolling pin, then roll out dough on lightly rice-floured board to 1/2 inch thick. Cut out with floured doughnut cutter. Fry in deep hot fat at 375 F. Turn doughnuts as they rise to surface. Fry until brown on both sides. Drain on absorbent paper. Cool and dust with granulated or gluten-free icing sugar. Makes 1 1/2 dozen.

DOUGHNUTS

tried
makes 16 donuts

2 eggs
1/2 cup sugar
1 tsp vanilla
2 tbsp melted margarine

1 1/4 cups rice flour
1/2 cup potato starch flour
2 1/2 tsp baking powder
1/4 tsp nutmeg
1/2 tsp cinnamon

Beat eggs, add sugar and vanilla, then beat well until thick. Sift flours and mix with other dry ingredients. Add egg mixture all at once to the dry ingredients. Chill well. Roll out on a lightly rice- floured board until 1/2 inch thick. Cut with doughnut cutter. Fry in deep fat at 375 F. Turn doughnuts as they rise to surface. Fry until golden brown on both sides. Drain on absorbent paper. Cool and dust with granulated sugar.

FRITTERS

1/4 cup white rice flour
1/4 cup brown rice flour
1/2 cup potato flour
1 tbsp sugar
1/2 tsp salt
2 tsp baking powder

2 eggs
3 tbsp oil or melted margarine
3/8 cup milk

Mix as for pancakes by sifting all dry ingredients into a large bowl. Beat eggs and combine with melted margarine and milk. Add all at once to dry ingredients. Spoon batter into hot deep fat and fry as for doughnuts.

Fritters may be used for a luncheon or supper food, and fruit fritters are a change for dessert. The batter may be used to coat larger pieces of fruit, or chopped fruit, corn, fish and meat may be folded into the batter. An extra 1 tbsp sugar may be added to the fritter batter.

GLUTEN FREE ANYTIME

APPLE FRITTERS

Peel and core apples and cut into thick slices. Each slice
may be sprinkled with gluten-free icing sugar and lemon
juice before dipping into the batter, or the apple slices can
be dipped directly into the batter. Coat the fruit well. Fry
in deep fat at 375 F and continue as directed for doughnuts,
drain on paper towels, and sprinkle with gluten-free icing
sugar. Serve hot. Apples may be chopped and added to the
fritter batter before deep frying.

BANANA FRITTERS

Peel and cut bananas into 1/2 inch thick pieces. Dip in
orange juice while preparing the fritter batter. Prepare as
for apple fritters.

CORN FRITTERS

Using the basic batter, add 1/2 tsp more salt and a dash of
pepper to the dry ingredients. Fold in 1 cup of drained
kernel corn. Fry like a thick pancake in deep fat (approximately 1/2 inch)in a heavy fry pan at medium heat (350 F)
until golden brown and cooked through.

MEAT, FISH FRITTERS

Using the basic batter, if desired add 1/4 tsp paprika, a little chopped parsley, and 1/4 tsp onion salt to the dry ingredients. Fold in 3/4 cup meat or fish. Fry as before. Serve with a cheese or cream sauce that has chopped hard cooked egg or sauteed mushrooms added.

* Note: Meat, fish, or corn fritters may be fried in deep fat (at least 3 inches deep). Spoon out the batter into hot fat. Fry from 5 - 8 minutes to cook through.

PANCAKES OR WAFFLES

1/4 cup white rice flour
1/4 cup brown rice flour
1/2 cup potato starch
1 tbsp sugar
1/2 tsp salt
2 tsp baking powder

2 eggs
3 tbsp oil or melted margarine
1/2 cup milk (or more depending on desired consistency)

Mix together the dry ingredients. Then add milk, eggs, and oil mixture to the dry ingredients and beat until smooth. Fry first batch on lightly greased hot skillet. Can use cold pancakes as bread for sandwiches.

WAFFLES - Follow above recipe adding 1/4 cup more milk for a more liquid consistency. Pour batter into lightly greased hot waffle iron and cook until brown.

TRAVEL PANCAKE OR READY PANCAKE MIX FOR HOME

From above recipe mix together dry ingredients and store in ziplock bag in refrigerator if possible. When you are ready for your camping breakfast - measure out 1/2 cup of dry mixture, add 1 egg, 1 1/2 tbsp oil, and 1/4 cup milk. Beat until smooth and prepare as above. You have a quick pancake breakfast.

Makes 4 medium pancakes.

FLUFFY APPLE PANCAKES

2 - 3 medium apples
1/4 cup butter or margarine
1/4 cup white rice flour
1/4 cup potato starch
1/4 tsp salt

3 egg yolks
3/4 cup light cream (canned 2% evaporated
milk can be used)
2 tbsp cooled, melted butter or margarine
3 egg whites at room temperature
pinch cream of tartar
1 tbsp sugar
2 tsp butter or margarine

Set oven to 350. Cut apples into thin wedges, core; peel if desired. Saute quickly in the 1/4 cup margarine until crisp tender. Remove from pan.

Combine flours, salt, cream into mixing bowl. Beat in egg yolks, one at a time, add 2 tbsp melted margarine.
In another bowl, beat egg whites with cream of tartar until soft peaks; beat in sugar and beat until stiff peaks form.
Fold into egg yolk batter using rubber spatula.

Heat the 2 tsp margarine in a heavy 10 inch frying pan that can be placed in an oven. Remove from heat and pour batter into pan. Arrange apple wedges over batter. Bake at 350 until pancake is set - about 20 minutes. Put under broiler for a few seconds until top is golden. Serve immediately in wedges with maple syrup or other fruit syrups. Makes 4 - 8 servings depending on use, breakfast or lunch.

Pancake Tips: For children, pancake batter may be shaped into bunnies and other animals as you pour the batter onto the griddle.

BUCKWHEAT PANCAKES

3/4 cup buckwheat
1/2 cup potato starch
1/2 cup brown rice flour
2 1/2 tsp baking powder
1/2 tsp salt
1/2 tsp baking soda

1 1/4 cups buttermilk or 1 cup sour milk
2 tbsp cooking oil
2 eggs

Sift, measure, and mix together the flours, then sift all dry
ingredients together into bowl. Beat eggs with buttermilk
and oil. Add all at once to dry ingredients and blend. Let
stand for 1 - 2 hours if possible. Cook on hot griddle.
Pancakes if not too large, can be toasted. Store extras well
sealed in refrigerator.

POTATO PANCAKES

2 medium size potatoes about 12 oz, peeled
1 tbsp lemon juice, freshly squeezed if
desired
1/4 cup margarine, melted
2 tbsp "Gluten Free Anytime" Mix
1/8 - 1/4 cup finely grated onion
1 large egg, beaten
1/2 tsp salt
1/4 tsp black pepper
1 tbsp chopped fresh or 1 tsp dried parsley
(optional)
1/4 tsp baking powder
1 tbsp vegetable oil, as needed
1 tbsp margarine, as needed

Grate potatoes in large bowl, then toss with lemon juice to
coat thoroughly, and let stand 5 minutes. Drain well.

Add melted margarine, flour, onion, egg, salt, pepper and
baking powder to potatoes, then stir to mix well. In a large
skillet over medium heat, heat 1 tbsp each of oil and
margarine. Spoon potato mixture into the skillet, using fork
to flatten each portion into thin rounds about 2 1/2 inch.
Cook pancakes 3 to 4 minutes on each side until golden
brown and cooked through. Remove to paper towels to
drain, keeping warm in 300 F oven. Serve immediately.
Makes about 16 pancakes.

CREPES

1 cup sifted white rice flour 1/4 tsp salt
1 tbsp sugar (optional)

3 eggs
1 cup milk
2 tbsp melted butter or margarine

Sift together flour, salt, (and sugar if used). Beat in eggs, milk and melted butter until very smooth and free from lumps about 2 - 3 minutes. (a blender may be used, scrape down sides after a minute of blending). Let chill for 2 hours, covered, before cooking. The crepe batter can be used immediately, but batter improves with standing. Heat a crepe pan or 7 inch frying pan until a few drops of water dance over the surface of the pan. Immediately butter the pan, pour about 1/4 cup of batter onto pan, quickly rotating pan to make the batter cover the entire surface. With a wide spatula gently lift an edge to see if the bottom is golden. The top will look dry (This takes only a few minutes). Slide the crepe or turn it over onto waxed paper. Crepes do not need to be browned on both sides.

Stack crepes with wax paper between them, not more than 6 or 7 to a pile. Refrigerate, well wrapped or freeze if not needed immediately. Makes approximately 12 crepes.

Crepes may be used for the main course or a desssert.

<u>For Main Course</u>

A) Make a thick white (cream) sauce:
      1/4 cup butter or margarine
      1 cup milk
      4 tbsp brown or white rice flour
            (or 2 tbsps corn starch)
      1/4 tsp salt
      Fresh ground pepper

Melt butter and add the flour (cornstarch is mixed with the cold milk and then poured into the melted butter). Add milk, stir over medium heat until thickened. Add seasonings.

For a cheese sauce add 1/2 cup grated cheddar cheese to the thickened white sauce and heat until melted. Sliced mushrooms or chopped hard cooked egg can also be added for variety. If mushrooms are added, they can be omitted from the filling mixture.

B) Filling:
>1/4 cup chopped onions
>1/2 cup sliced mushrooms
>2 tbsp butter
>1/4 cup chopped green pepper (opt)
>1/2 tsp salt
>2 cups diced ham, chicken, fish
>pepper to taste

Saute onions, and mushrooms (also green pepper if used) in the 2 tbsp butter. Add the meat, poultry, or fish and heat through. Season to taste. Add 3/4 cup sauce to filling and stir together gently.

To complete the crepes, place 2 tbsp of filling in the center of a crepe. Fold side edges to center of crepe over the filling and fold up bottom edge and top edge over like an envelope. Place folded crepes in a greased baking dish. Top with remainder of the sauce and sprinkle with chopped parsley. Bake at 350 for about 1/2 hour.

ANOTHER CREAM SAUCE

3/4 cup salad dressing
3 1/2 tbsp white rice flour
1/2 tsp salt
dash pepper
1 1/2 cup milk
3/4 cup grated cheddar or Swiss Cheese

Combine salad dressing, rice flour and seasonings. Gradually add milk. Cook over medium heat, stirring constantly until thickened. Add cheese and stir until melted.

DESSERT CREPES

Fast and easy: 2 tbsp canned pie filling can be spooned on each crepe, rolled up and topped with whipped cream.

FRUIT CREPE

Heat 2 cups fruit (blueberries, cherries) with 1 tsp cinnamon, and 2 tbsp sugar. Cover and cook for 5 minutes. Strain fruit, reserving sauce. Spoon 2 tbsp fruit on each crepe, roll up and spoon the sauce over which has been mixed with 3/4 cup yogurt.

BASIC COOKIES

1/2 cup shortening
3/4 cup brown sugar
2 eggs, beaten
1 tsp vanilla

1 cup white rice flour
1/2 tsp baking soda
1/2 tsp salt
1/2 cup nuts, raisins or chocolate chips
(optional)

Preheat oven to 350 F. Grease cookie sheet. Cream shortening with sugar, then add eggs and vanilla and mix well. Mix in sifted dry ingredients, then add nuts, raisins, or chocolate chips. Drop on greased cookie sheet. Bake for 10 - 15 minutes.

<u>APPLE NUT COOKIES</u>

1/2 cup margarine
1 cup brown sugar
1 egg
1/4 cup apple juice
1 1/2 cups rice flour
1/2 cup soya flour
1/2 tsp baking powder
1 tsp baking soda
1/4 tsp salt
1 tsp cinnamon
1/2 tsp each allspice & cloves
1/2 cup chopped walnuts
2 apples, peeled, cored, shredded

Preheat oven to 400 F. Sift dry ingredients together. Set aside. Cream margarine, then add sugar and cream together well. Beat in egg. Add dry ingredients alternately with apple juice. Add apples and nuts and mix until well blended. Drop by the teaspoonful onto ungreased cookie sheets. Bake at 400 F for 10 - 12 minutes. Makes about 3 1/2 dozen cookies.

These cookies may be glazed with a mixture of 1 cup gluten-free icing sugar mixed with 1 tbsp apple juice or more depending on dryness of sugar.

ROLLED OUT SUGAR COOKIES

3/4 cup butter or margarine
3/4 cup brown sugar
3/4 cup white sugar
2 eggs
2 tsp vanilla

1 cup white rice flour
1 cup soya flour
1/2 cup potato starch
2 tsp baking powder
1/2 tsp salt

Preheat oven to 350 F. Sift together flours, starch, baking powder and salt, then set aside. Cream butter, add sugars gradually and cream well. Beat in vanilla and eggs. Stir in sifted dry ingredients. Cover and chill 3 hours. Roll out on lightly floured board (use rice flour). Cut out cookies. Bake on ungreased cookie sheets 8 - 10 minutes or until lightly browned. Remove from pan immediately. Makes about 3 dozen cookies depending on size of cutters.

Variation: To dry ingredients add 1/4 cup cocoa and 1/2 cup chopped nuts and follow instructions above. Shape dough in long roll, chill for 2 hours, then slice with sharp knife 1/4 inch thick, and bake at 350 for 12 - 15 minutes.

CHOCOLATE CHIP COOKIES

1/2 cup brown sugar
1/4 cup white sugar
1 egg
1 tsp vanilla
1/2 cup + 2 tbsp margarine

1/2 cup potato starch
1 cup soya flour
3/4 tsp baking soda
1/2 tsp baking powder
1/2 tsp salt
1/2 cup chopped walnuts
1/2 cup semi-sweet chocolate chips

Heat oven to 375 F. Grease baking sheets. Sift together flours, salt, baking powder, and baking soda, then set aside. Cream margarine, add sugars and blend well. Beat in vanilla and egg. Stir in sifted dry ingredients, chocolate chips, and nuts. Bake at 375 F for 10 - 12 minutes. Makes about 3 dozen cookies.

GINGER SNAPS

1/4 cup margarine
1/2 cup sugar
1 egg
1/8 cup molasses

1 tsp baking soda
1/2 cup soya flour
1/4 cup cornstarch
1/4 cup potato starch
1/4 tsp ginger
1/2 tsp cinnamon
1/4 tsp salt

Preheat oven to 350 F and grease cookie sheets. Mix molasses and baking soda. Cream margarine and sugar. Add molasses mixture. Beat in egg. Stir in sifted dry ingredients and mix well. Spoon onto greased cookie sheets or pinch off bits of dough and roll in sugar. Bake at 350 F for 10 - 12 minutes.

PUMPKIN COOKIES

1 cup sugar
1/2 cup shortening
1 cup pumpkin
1 tsp vanilla

1/2 tsp salt
1 cup rice flour
3/4 cup potato starch
1 tsp baking soda
1 tsp baking powder
1 tsp cinnamon
1 cup raisins
1/2 cup nuts

Preheat oven to 350 F. Cream shortening, vanilla, and sugar. Add sifted dry ingredients, blend to mix. Add pumpkin, raisins, and nuts. Drop onto ungreased cookie sheets. Bake for 10 minutes.

DAD'S COOKIES

1/2 cup margarine or butter
1/2 cup white sugar
1/4 cup brown sugar, packed
1 egg
1 tsp vanilla

1/2 cup rice flour
1/4 cup potato starch
1/2 tsp baking soda
1/2 tsp baking powder
1/2 cup coconut
1/2 cup + 2 tbsp rolled rice
1/4 tsp salt

Cream together margarine and sugars. Add the egg and mix well. Stir in coconut, vanilla, and rolled rice. Sift, measure, then sift together flours, baking powder, baking soda, and salt. Add to creamed mixture and mix well. Let sit for 1/2 hour. Heat oven to 350 F and grease cookie sheets. Roll into small balls. Press down with fork or back of glass dipped in granulated sugar. Place on baking sheet with 2 inches between. Bake at 350 F for 8 - 10 minutes.

DATE COCONUT BALLS

1/4 cup margarine
8 oz dates, chopped
1 cup sugar
1 egg

2 cups toasted gluten-free rice cereal
1/4 cup chopped nuts
coconut

Combine margarine, dates, sugar, and egg in a saucepan over medium heat until the margarine melts and mixture thickens. Place the cereal and nuts in a mixing bowl and pour the date mixture over. Blend. Cool slightly. Shape into ball and roll in coconut. Place on baking sheets lined with waxed paper and let remain on the sheets for 3 hours. Then place balls in a container separated by sheets of waxed paper. Freezes well. Yields 3 dozen.

FRYING PAN COOKIES

1 egg
1 cup brown sugar

3/4 cup chopped dates
3/4 cup coconut
1/4 cup chopped walnuts
1 tsp vanilla
1/8 tsp salt
additional coconut

Beat egg, add sugar, and remaining ingredients. Stir well. Put mixture into greased frying pan and simmer, stirring frequently for about 20 minutes. Mixture should be thick. Cool to lukewarm. Shape into small logs and roll in additional coconut. Chill.

POPPY SEED COOKIES

1/2 cup margarine or butter
1/2 cup granulated sugar
1 egg, beaten
1 tbsp yogurt or sour cream

1/2 cup soya flour
1/2 cup cornstarch
1/2 cup white rice flour
1/2 tsp baking powder
1/4 tsp baking soda
pinch of salt
1/4 cup poppy seeds
1/2 cup coconut

Cream butter, beat in sugar until light and fluffy. Blend in egg and yogurt/sour cream. Sift together flours, cornstarch, baking powder, baking soda, and salt. Stir in poppy seed. Add this mixture to the creamed mixture and mix well. Add coconut. Chill 1 hour. Preheat oven to 375 F. Grease cookie sheets. Form into 1 inch balls and place on baking sheets. Bake for 8 - 10 minutes. Let cool on rack.

<u>MACAROONS</u>

(Have egg whites at room temperature for best volume)
2 egg whites
2/3 cup fine granulated sugar
1 tsp vanilla
1/8 tsp cream of tartar
1/4 tsp salt
1 cup coconut

Preheat oven to 325 F. Cover a baking sheet with unglazed brown paper. Beat egg whites and cream of tartar until just stiff enough to hold a soft peak. Gradually add sugar and salt, beating after each addition until whites form a firmer peak. Fold in vanilla and coconut. Drop by spoonfuls onto the baking sheet 1 1/2 inches apart. Bake at 325 F for about 30 minutes. Remove from the paper immediately and cool on rack. Makes about 2 1/2 dozen.

CHOCOLATE MACAROONS

2 egg whites
3 tbsp cocoa
1/4 tsp salt
1/4 tsp cream of tartar
3/4 cup granulated sugar

1 cup coconut
1 cup puffed rice, either whole brown puffed rice or white puffed rice
1/2 cup chopped pecans
1 tsp vanilla

Preheat oven to 300 F. Cover baking sheets with brown paper. Grease paper. Beat egg whites until just stiff enough to hold soft peaks. Sift cocoa, salt and sugar together and add gradually a tablespoon at a time to the egg whites and beat until a soft peak is formed. Fold in vanilla, rice cereal, coconut and nuts. Drop by spoonfuls onto prepared pans. Bake at 300 F for 35 - 40 minutes. Remove immediately from paper and cool on wire rack.

OLD FASHIONED PEANUT BUTTER COOKIES

1/2 cup butter
1/2 cup peanut butter
1/2 cup brown sugar
1/2 cup granulated sugar
1 egg

1/2 cup soya flour
1/2 cup brown rice flour
1/2 cup + 2 tbsp potato starch
1/2 tsp baking powder
1 tsp baking soda
1/4 tsp salt

Sift flours, potato starch, baking soda, baking powder and salt together; set aside. Cream butter, peanut butter, and sugar together very well. Beat in egg mixing well. Add dry ingredients to creamed mixture. Mix well. Chill. Preheat oven to 375 F. Shape dough into 1 inch balls and place 2 inches apart on ungreased baking sheets. Press flat with floured fork. Bake for approximately 15 minutes. Yields about 36 cookies.

BASIC REFRIGERATOR COOKIES

3 cups "Gluten Free Anytime" Mix
2 tsp baking powder
1/2 tsp baking soda
1/4 tsp salt

1/2 cup margarine or butter
1/2 cup shortening
1 cup granulated sugar
2 eggs
2 tsp vanilla

Sift mix, then sift all dry ingredients together except sugar. Cream margarine, shortening and sugar together until fluffy. Add eggs and vanilla and blend well. Stir flour mixture into creamed mixture. Blend well. Chill at least 1/2 hour. Shape dough into 2 rolls about 1 1/2 inches in diameter. Wrap in waxed paper and chill overnight until firm to the touch. Preheat oven to 375 F. Slice with a sharp knife into thin slices. Place on ungreased cookie sheets and bake about 10 minutes. Remove from cookie sheets to cool.

GLUTEN FREE ANYTIME

Variations

<u>Butternut</u> - Substitute 1 cup brown sugar (packed) for the 1 cup granulated sugar. Mix in 1/2 cup chopped pecans.

<u>Orange</u> - To the basic recipe add 1 tbsp finely grated orange rind and 1 tbsp orange juice to the creamed mixture.

<u>Chocolate</u> - To the basic recipe add 2 squares unsweetened chocolate, melted and cooled, to the creamed mixture. 1/2 cup chopped nuts also may be added.

For quick chilling, put rolls in freezer for an hour. Use a sharp, thin-bladed knife for slicing cookies. Cut straight down through roll, do not use a sawing motion.

Refrigerator doughs keep well in the refrigerator for a few weeks. Slice and bake as needed.

CINNAMON ROUNDS

1/2 cup margarine
1 cup granulated sugar
1 egg, beaten
1 tsp vanilla

1/2 cup brown rice flour
1/2 cup potato starch
1/4 cup soya flour
1 1/2 tsp baking powder
1/4 tsp salt
2 tsp cinnamon
1/2 cup finely chopped nuts

Preheat oven to 375 F. Grease baking sheets. Cream margarine and sugar together. Add egg and vanilla and blend well. Sift together flours, starch, baking powder, salt and 1 tsp cinnamon. Add to creamed mixture. Mold the mixture using about 1 tbsp into balls and roll in a mixture of the chopped nuts and remaining 1 tsp cinnamon. Place on prepared baking sheets about 2 inches apart. Bake for 15 minutes. Remove immediately from baking sheets. Yields about 2 1/2 dozen.

SPICE DATE COOKIES

1/4 cup shortening
3/4 cup brown sugar
1/2 tsp vanilla
1 egg, well beaten

3/4 cup soya flour
1/2 cup potato starch
1/2 tsp baking soda
3/4 tsp baking powder
1/4 tsp salt
1/4 tsp cinnamon
1/8 tsp nutmeg
1/2 cup sour cream or yogurt
1 cup chopped, pitted dates

Preheat oven to 400 F. Grease baking sheets. Cream shortening, brown sugar, and vanilla. Add egg, and mix well.
Sift together dry ingredients. Add to creamed mixture
alternately with yogurt or sour cream. Stir in dates. Drop
from teaspoon about 2 inches apart onto prepared cookie
sheets. Bake in the hot oven about 10 minutes. Cool
slightly before removing from pan. Yields approximately
3 1/2 dozen.

GINGERBREAD COOKIES

1/2 cup shortening
1/2 cup sugar
1/2 cup molasses
1 egg

1 cup soya flour
1/2 cup potato starch
1 cup white rice flour
1 1/2 tsp baking powder
1/2 tsp baking soda
1 tsp cloves
1 tsp ginger
1 tsp cinnamon
1/2 tsp salt

Grease cookie sheets. Cream shortening, sugar, and molasses. Add egg. Sift dry ingredients together, and add to creamed mixture. Chill well. Preheat oven to 350 F. Roll out on rice-floured board. Cut in desired shape. Bake for 10 - 12 minutes.

TANGY ORANGE DROP COOKIES

1/2 cup margarine (part shortening)
3/4 cup sugar
1 egg

3/4 cup soya flour
3/4 cup potato starch
1 1/2 tsp baking powder
1/2 tsp salt
3 tbsp orange juice
1 tsp grated orange rind
1/2 cup raisins (optional)

Preheat oven to 350 F. Grease baking sheets. Cream margarine, shortening, and sugar until fluffy. Add egg and beat well. Add orange rind. Sift dry ingredients together, then stir in alternately with orange juice. Blend in raisins if used. Drop by spoonfuls onto prepared pans leaving 2 inches between cookies. Bake for about 15 minutes.

SHORTBREAD

1/2 lb butter
1/2 cup gluten free icing sugar
1 tsp vanilla or almond flavoring
1 cup white rice flour
1 cup cornstarch

Preheat oven to 325 F.

Whip butter until creamy and white. Add icing sugar and beat in well. Whip in flavoring. Sift cornstarch and rice flour together and then blend into the butter mixture.

Roll into 1 inch balls and flatten with a fork dipped in gluten free icing sugar. Bake on ungreased baking sheet for 20 - 25 minutes. Let cool, then remove shortbread. Store in an airtight container. These cookies freeze well.

EASY BROWNIES

1/2 cup margarine
2 oz unsweetened chocolate

1 cup sugar
2 eggs
1 tsp vanilla
1/2 cup "Gluten Free Anytime" Mix
3/4 cup chopped nuts
1 1/2 tsp baking powder
pinch salt

Preheat oven to 350 F. Grease a 9 inch square pan.

In a microwave - safe measuring cup (4 cup size), melt margarine and chocolate together on HI for about 1 - 2 minutes. Remove from microwave and stir in sugar; the baking mix, salt and baking powder which have been mixed together, and vanilla. Beat in eggs one at a time. Blend well. Pour into the prepared pan and bake for about 30 minutes. Cool in pan before cutting.

<u>BUTTERSCOTCH BROWNIES</u>

1/4 cup margarine
1 cup brown sugar
1/2 tsp vanilla
1 egg

1/2 cup rice flour
1 tsp baking powder
1/2 tsp salt
1/2 cup chopped nuts

Preheat oven to 350 F and grease 8 inch square pan.. Sift together dry ingredients and set aside.

Melt margarine over low heat, remove from heat and stir in sugar until blended. Cool. Stir in egg. Blend in dry ingredients. Add vanilla and nuts. Spoon into pan. Bake for approximately 25 minutes. Cut into bars while warm.

ZUCCHINI CINNAMON BROWNIES

1/3 cup soft margarine
1 cup brown sugar
1/2 tsp vanilla
1 egg

1/2 tsp salt
1/4 tsp nutmeg
1 1/2 tsp cinnamon
1/4 tsp baking powder
1 cup brown rice flour and soya mixed
1/2 cup chopped nuts
1 cup chopped zucchini

Preheat oven to 350 F. Grease a 9 inch square pan.

Cream margarine, sugar, egg, and vanilla. Beat well. Add
mixed dry ingredients and stir. Add zucchini and nuts.
Bake for 30 - 35 minutes.

Jasy loves this!

PEANUT BUTTER BROWNIES

1/2 cup margarine
1/2 cup peanut butter either smooth or
crunchy (gluten-free)
1 cup brown sugar, packed
1 tsp vanilla
2 eggs

1/2 cup soya flour
1/2 cup potato starch
1 1/2 tsp baking powder
1/4 tsp salt
1 cup semi-sweet chocolate chips

Preheat oven to 350 F. Grease a 9 inch square cake pan.

Cream together margarine and peanut butter, gradually add sugar, continue to beat until fluffy. Beat in eggs, one at a time. Add vanilla. Sift dry ingredients together and add to creamed mixture stirring to blend. Fold in chocolate chips. Spread in prepared pan and bake 30 - 35 minutes. Cool in pan, then cut into bars or squares. Makes 24 brownies.

SAUCEPAN GUMDROP BARS

1/2 cup margarine or butter
1/3 cup brown sugar
1/3 cup granulated sugar
2 tbsp water

1/2 cup soya flour
1/2 cup potato starch
1 1/2 tsp baking powder
1/4 tsp salt
1 egg
1 tsp vanilla
2/3 cup small baking gumdrops, finely cut

Preheat oven to 350 F. Grease a 9 inch square pan.

Melt margarine in saucepan or in a pyrex glass bowl in microwave. Remove from heat. Add sugars and water. Blend. Stir in dry ingredients; add egg and vanilla beaten well. Stir in gumdrops. Pour into prepared pan and bake for 30 minutes. Do not overbake. Cool and then cut into bars.

QUICK SQUARES

1/2 cup butter
1 cup brown sugar
2 eggs
1 tsp vanilla
1 cup "Gluten Free Anytime" Mix
1/2 tsp salt
1/4 tsp baking powder
1/2 cup chocolate chips

Preheat oven to 350 F and grease 8 x 8 inch pan. Cream butter with sugar. Add eggs and vanilla, beat well. Add sifted dry ingredients to creamed mixture. Blend, add chocolate chips. Bake in prepared pan for 20 - 25 minutes. Cool and cut into squares.

PUFFED BROWN RICE CAKE

Rice Krispie Puffed Squares

1/2 cup butter
1 cup Rogers syrup
1 cup brown sugar
2 tsp cocoa
2 tsp vanilla

Stir all ingredients in a saucepan and just bring to a boil. Pour over 8 cups of puffed rice and pack in a buttered 9 inch pan. Let partly set, then mark into squares.

RASPBERRY DREAM BARS

Base: 3/4 cup soya flour
3/4 cup potato starch
3/4 tsp baking powder
1/4 tsp salt
1/2 cup butter (part shortening)
1 egg, slightly beaten
1/3 cup brown sugar

Topping:
1 cup brown sugar
2 tbsp white rice flour
1 tsp baking powder
1/4 tsp salt
2 eggs
1/2 tsp vanilla
1/2 cup coconut
1/2 cup chopped walnuts
1/2 cup raspberry jam

Preheat oven to 425 F. Grease a 9 inch square pan.

Sift soya flour, potato starch, baking powder, and salt together. Cut in the butter and shortening until mixture is crumbly. Add slightly beaten egg and sugar; mix thoroughly. Pat mixture into prepared pan. Bake for 10 minutes. Remove from oven; then reduce heat to 350 F. Combine brown sugar, flour, baking powder, and salt. Set aside. Beat eggs and stir in the dry ingredients, vanilla, coconut, and nuts. Carefully spread jam over the partially baked crust. Spoon the coconut-nut mixture on top and spread evenly. Bake at 350 F for 25 minutes. Cool. Cut in bars.

MATRIMONIAL SQUARES

1 cup chopped dates
1/2 cup boiling water
2 tbsp brown sugar
1 tsp lemon juice

1/2 cup butter or margarine
1/2 cup brown sugar
1 tsp vanilla
1/2 cup potato starch
1/2 cup soya flour
1 cup corn germ
1/8 tsp salt
1/2 tsp baking soda

For filling: cook dates, water and brown sugar until soft.
Cool and add lemon juice. Preheat oven to 350 F. Grease a
9 x 9 inch pan. Cream butter and sugar and blend in vanilla. Sift together potato starch, soya flour, salt and baking
soda. Mix in corn germ. Add to creamed mixture, rubbing
together to form a crumb mixture. Press half of mixture
into a greased pan (an egg turner works well). Spread with
date mixture. Sprinkle the remaining crumbs over the dates
and press in gently. Bake for 25 minutes. When cool, cut
into squares.

BASIC CAKE

2 cups "Gluten Free Anytime" Mix
4 tsp baking powder
1/2 tsp salt
3/4 cup milk

1 tsp vanilla
1 tsp lemon extract
3 eggs
1/2 cup margarine
1 cup sugar

Preheat oven to 350 F. Grease a 9 inch square cake pan.

Cream margarine well, gradually add sugar and beat until fluffy. Add eggs one at a time beating well after each addition. Add flavorings. Sift dry ingredients together and add alternately with the milk adding flour first and last. Blend well. Spoon into prepared pan and bake at 350 F approximately 45 minutes.

Variations:
1. Orange - add 2 tbsp grated orange rind to the creamed mixture. Use 1/2 cup orange juice and 1/4 cup milk in place of the 3/4 cup milk.

2. Chocolate - melt 2 squares unsweetened chocolate and add after the eggs are blended in. Reduce milk to 1/2 cup.

3. Spice - Add 1 tsp cinnamon, 1/2 tsp each cloves and nutmeg to the dry ingredients, 1/2 cup raisins or nuts may be added by folding in to the finished batter. Use a broiled topping for icing.

PINEAPPLE UPSIDE DOWN CAKE

Melt 1/4 cup margarine in a deep 9 inch square cake pan over direct heat or in the oven (if using glass pan this may be done in a microwave on high for 1 minute). Tip pan to distribute melted butter evenly, sprinkle with 1/2 cup brown sugar. Cover with a layer of drained pineapple rings. Drop a maraschino cherry into easy ring. Pour prepared cake batter over the fruit and bake as for basic cake. Cool 5 minutes and invert. Serve warm with whipped dessert topping.
  * Use canned drained peach halves cut side down for variety *

RHUBARB CAKE PUDDING

Melt 1/3 cup butter in 9 x 9 inch pan. Sprinkle melted butter with 1 cup brown sugar, 4 cups cut-up rhubarb, 1 tbsp grated orange rind. Proceed as for pineapple upside down cake. Serve warm with whipped cream.

CHOCOLATE SOUR CREAM CAKE

3 eggs
1 cup thick sour cream
1 1/4 cups sugar
1 tsp vanilla
1/4 cup hot water
2 - 1 oz squares unsweetened chocolate

1 cup white rice flour
1/2 cup potato starch
1/4 cup soya flour
1/2 tsp baking powder
1 tsp baking soda
1/2 tsp salt
pinch cream of tartar

Preheat oven to 350 F. Grease a 7 x 11 or 9 inch square pan. Melt chocolate in the hot water over low heat. Cool. Separate eggs. Beat egg yolks, add cream and beat. Gradually add the sugar and beat until thick. Add the chocolate mixture and vanilla to the egg-cream mixture. Stir in sifted dry ingredients except cream of tartar. Beat egg whites with cream of tartar. Fold in stiffly beaten egg whites. Pour into pan and bake for 45 - 50 minutes.
(1 tsp peppermint flavoring may be added instead of the vanilla to make a chocolate peppermint cake)

SURPRISE CHOCOLATE CAKE

3/4 cup margarine
1 cup brown sugar
3/4 cup white sugar
4 eggs
2 tsp vanilla
1 cup soya flour
1 cup white rice flour
1/2 cup potato starch
4 tsp baking powder
2 tsp baking soda
1 tsp each salt & cinnamon
1 tsp unflavored gelatin
1/2 tsp nutmeg
1/2 cup cocoa
1 cup chopped walnuts (opt)
1/2 cup buttermilk or sour milk
2 cups peeled and grated zucchini

Preheat oven to 350 F. Grease a 9 x 13 pan or a 25 cm tube
pan.
Combine flours, cocoa, baking powder, baking soda, salt,
unflavored gelatin, spices in a medium bowl. Set aside.
Beat margarine and sugars until well creamed together.
Add vanilla, and eggs beating well. Stir in zucchini. Stir in
sifted dry ingredients alternately with milk. Add nuts last if

used. Blend. Spoon into prepared pan and bake for 45 - 50 minutes for 9 x 13 pan, or 60 - 70 minutes for tube pan or until cake springs back when lightly touched.
Cool in pan 15 minutes and turn out if using a tube pan and leave in the 9 x 13 inch pan. Frost as desired. (Better the second day)

BANANA CAKE

1/3 cup margarine
1 cup white sugar
1 tsp vanilla
2 eggs
1 tsp lemon extract
1 1/2 cups white rice flour
1/2 cup potato starch
3 tsp baking powder
1/2 tsp baking soda
1/2 tsp salt
1 1/4 cups mashed ripe bananas
1/3 cup buttermilk or sour milk

Preheat oven to 350 F. Grease 8 or 9 inch cake pan. Cream butter well, sugar, add flavorings until fluffy. Beat in eggs one at a time, blending well after each addition. Sift dry ingredients together and add alternately with bananas and milk. Pour in prepared pan and bake 45 minutes.

DUTCH APPLE CAKE

1/2 cup margarine
3/4 cup sugar
2 eggs
1 tsp lemon extract
4 oz (1/2 cup) milk

1 cup white rice flour
1/3 cup cornstarch
1 3/4 tsp baking powder
dash salt
2 apples, peeled and sliced

Preheat oven to 375 F, grease and rice flour a 9 inch round cake pan. Cream margarine, sugar, lemon extract, and eggs. Add sifted dry ingredients, alternately with milk and mix well together. Pour batter into prepared pan. Set apples on top of batter. Sprinkle with mixture of sugar and cinnamon over apples (approximately 1/4 cup sugar & 1 tsp cinnamon). Bake at 375 F for 45 - 50 minutes. Cool in pan for 20 minutes.

ANGEL FOOD CAKE

8 egg whites
1 tsp cream of tartar
1/4 tsp salt
1 1/4 cup fine granulated sugar

1 tsp vanilla
1/2 tsp almond flavoring
3/4 cup potato starch
1/4 cup rice flour

Preheat oven to 375 F. Sift flour with 1/4 cup sugar, 4 times. Beat egg whites until frothy, add cream of tartar, salt, and beat until soft peaks form. Add remaining 1 cup sugar, 1 tbsp at a time beating until whites stand in stiff peaks. Fold in flavoring and flour-sugar mixture 1/4 of it at a time.

Pour into ungreased 10 inch tube pan. Gently cut through batter with knife to remove air spaces. Bake at 375 F for 40 minutes. Don't invert cake for about 10 - 15 minutes. Cut around edges and under bottom section before turning out onto a plate. Cut when cool with a serrated knife, moistened in warm water.

GOLD CAKE
(To use the 8 egg yolks from Angel Food Cake)
1 cup white rice flour
1/2 cup potato starch
1/2 tsp salt
4 tsp baking powder
1/8 tsp nutmeg
1/2 cup milk
8 egg yolks (2/3 cup)
1 cup sugar
6 tbsp margarine
1/2 tsp vanilla
1 tsp lemon juice & 1 tsp lemon rind

Line bottoms of 2 - 8 inch layer cake pans with waxed paper. Grease lightly. Set oven to 325 F. Sift dry ingredients together, except sugar. Set aside. Beat egg yolks until light and thick. Cream butter or margarine. Gradually add sugar and cream until smooth and fluffy. Add beaten egg yolks to creamed mixture and blend well. Beat in flavorings. Add dry ingredients alternately with milk, beginning and ending with flour and beat well after each addition. Pour into prepared pans. Bake in the slow oven for approximately 30 minutes. Cool 5 minutes in pan on rack and then turn out carefully on racks, removing the wax paper carefully. When cool, spread with a favorite filling or jelly, jam between layers; then ice with favorite frosting. The cake may be sprinkled with gluten-free icing sugar when barely cool.

SPONGE CAKE

3 eggs, separated
1/4 cup cold water
3/4 cup granulated sugar
1/4 tsp vanilla
1/4 tsp lemon extract
3/4 cup sifted potato starch
1/8 tsp salt
1/4 tsp cream of tartar

Preheat oven to 325 F. Grease and flour (with potato starch) a 9 inch layer pan. Beat egg yolks until thick and lemon colored, add water and beat until very thick. Gradually beat in sugar, then flavorings. Fold in starch sifted with salt, a little at a time. Beat egg whites until foamy, then add cream of tartar and beat until moist, stiff peaks form. Fold into egg yolk mixture. Pour into prepared pan and bake for 50 minutes. When slicing use a moistened knife. (a good cake for desserts like trifle, short cakes etc.)

try

CARROT AND PINEAPPLE CAKE

2/3 cup vegetable oil
2 eggs
1 tsp vanilla
3/4 cup sugar
1 1/2 cups rice flour
1 1/2 tsp baking powder
1 tsp baking soda
1 tsp cinnamon
1/2 tsp salt
1 cup shredded carrots
1/2 cup crushed pineapple with juice

Preheat oven to 350 F. Sift dry ingredients together. Add remaining ingredients and beat 2 minutes. Bake for 40 - 45 minutes in a greased 8 or 9 inch pan.

ORANGE DREAM CAKE

2/3 cup shortening
2 eggs
1/3 cup orange juice
1/3 cup water
2 tbsp lemon juice
1/4 tsp grated lemon rind
1 1/2 tsp grated orange rind

1 tsp salt
1 1/2 cups rice flour
1/2 cup potato starch
3 tsp baking powder
1/4 tsp baking soda
1 1/2 cups sugar

Preheat oven to 350 F. Line 2 - 8 inch layer pans with greased wax paper. Sift dry ingredients into mixing bowl. Drop in shortening. Add grated rinds, juices, and water. Beat 2 minutes at low speed. Add eggs; beat 2 more minutes. Add lemon juice and blend. Bake for approximately 30 minutes.

ORANGE CREAM FILLING

3 tsp grated orange rind
1/4 cup sugar
2 tbsp orange juice
1 cup coconut
1 cup heavy cream, whipped

Mix all ingredients except whipped cream; let stand for 15 minutes. Fold in cream. Frost cake layers.

APPLESAUCE CAKE

1/2 cup margarine
1 cup brown sugar
2 eggs
1 cup unsweetened applesauce
1/2 cup white rice flour
1/2 cup corn flour
1/2 cup tapioca starch
1 tsp baking soda
1 1/2 tsp baking powder
1/2 tsp salt
1/2 tsp cloves
1/2 tsp nutmeg
1 tsp cinnamon
1 cup raisins
1/2 cup chopped nuts (opt)

Preheat oven to 350 F. Grease an 8 x 8 inch square pan. Cream margarine and sugar well. Add eggs one at a time, beating well after each addition. Sift flours, starch, soda, baking powder, salt, and spices together. Add dry ingredients alternately with applesauce. Pour batter into prepared pan. Bake for approximately 40 - 45 minutes.

BEST EVER ORANGE CHIFFON CAKE

3/4 cup white rice flour
3/4 cup potato starch
1 1/2 cups granulated sugar
3 tsp baking powder
1 tsp salt
1/2 tsp unflavored gelatin
1/2 cup vegetable oil
7 egg yolks, unbeaten
1/2 cup orange juice
1/4 cup cold water
2 tbsp grated orange rind
1 cup egg whites (8)
1/2 tsp cream of tartar

Place oven rack at the lowest position.
Preheat oven to 325 F. Sift flour and starch, then sift
together with sugar, baking powder, salt, and unflavored
gelatin into a medium sized mixing bowl. Make a hollow
and add oil, egg yolks, juice, cold water and orange rind.
Mix with electric beater until smooth. Place egg whites
into large mixing bowl, add cream of tartar and beat until
very stiff peaks are formed. Pour egg yolk mixture over
beaten egg whites folding in gently until blended. Pour
into ungreased 10 x 4 inch tube pan and bake at 325 F for 1
hour; then increase temperature to 350 F and bake an
additional 10 - 15 minutes until the top springs back when

touched lightly. Turn pan upside down resting tube pan on a funnel or on the pan feet. Let cake cool completely before removing from pan.

VARIATIONS

<u>Chocolate Chiffon</u> - reduce rice flour to 1/2 cup and sift in 1/4 cup cocoa with the dry ingredients. Omit orange rind. Substitute 1/2 cup cold water for the 1/2 cup orange juice (total cold water now is 3/4 cup). The cake may be frosted with whipped cream or a chocolate glaze.

<u>Pineapple Chiffon</u> - Omit orange rind and substitute the 1/2 cup orange juice and 1/4 cup cold water with 3/4 cups unsweetened pineapple juice.

<u>Lemon Chiffon</u> - substitute the orange rind with 1 tbsp lemon rind and add 1 tsp lemon extract for flavoring. Omit the 1/2 cup orange juice and substitute it with 1/2 cup cold water.

The variations can be endless with a variety of flavorings eg. maple.

POUND CAKE

1 cup butter
1 cup berry sugar (fine granulated)
5 eggs
1 tsp vanilla extract
1 tsp almond extract

1 cup white rice flour
1/2 cup corn flour
1/2 cup potato starch
1 1/2 tsp baking powder
1/2 tsp salt
1 tsp unflavored gelatin

Preheat oven to 350 F. Grease a 9 x 5 inch loaf pan.

Cream butter, add sugar gradually and beat until very
fluffy. Add flavorings and blend. Add eggs one at a time
beating well after each addition. Sift dry ingredients together and add to the creamed mixture. Beat well. Pour
into prepared pan and bake for approximately 1 1/4 hours.
Cool in pan for 10 minutes before turning out. Cool completely before slicing.

ORANGE RAISIN CAKE

1/2 cup shortening
1 cup granulated sugar
1 tsp vanilla
2 eggs

1 cup white rice flour
1 cup potato starch
1 tsp baking powder
1 tsp baking soda
1/2 tsp salt
1 tbsp orange rind, grated
1/2 cup raisins, chopped
3/4 cup thick sour cream

Preheat oven to 350 F. Grease a 9 x 9 inch cake pan.
Cream shortening, gradually adding sugar and cream until
fluffy. Add vanilla, beat in eggs one at a time. Sift dry
ingredients together and add to creamed mixture. Blend
well, add orange rind and raisins. Add cream stirring only
until mixed. Bake 40 minutes or until done. Remove from
oven, cool 5 minutes, then pour a mixture of 1/2 cup sugar,
1 tsp grated orange rind and 1/2 cup orange juice over the
top of the cake.

SPICE CAKE

2 eggs separated
1/2 cup granulated sugar
1 1/4 cups white rice flour
1/2 cup potato starch
1/2 cup sweet rice flour
2 tsp baking powder
3/4 tsp baking soda
1 tsp salt
1 tsp cinnamon
3/4 tsp each cloves and nutmeg
1 cup brown sugar
1/3 cup vegetable oil
1 cup buttermilk
1/2 cup chocolate chips, raisins, or nuts (optional)

Preheat oven to 350 F. Grease well 2 round layer pans,
8 inch or 9 x 1 1/2 inch or an oblong pan 13 x 9 inch.
  Beat egg whites until frothy. Gradually beat in granulated
sugar and beat until very stiff and glossy.
  Sift flours, starch, baking powder, baking soda, salt and
spices in another mixing bowl. Add brown sugar, oil, and
2/3 of the buttermilk. Beat 1 minute medium speed on
mixer or quite vigorously by hand. Scrape sides and
bottom of bowl frequently. Add remaining buttermilk
and egg yolks. Beat 1 more minute. Fold in meringue.
Pour into prepared pans. Bake layers for 25 - 30 minutes,
oblong for 35 - 40 minutes.

UNCOOKED ICING

1 cold egg white
1 cup sugar
1/4 tsp cream of tartar
1/2 cup hot water
1 tsp vanilla

Beat until light and fluffy. (May be made ahead of time and stored in fridge - it does not need to harden)

BROILED FROSTING

1/4 cup margarine, melted
1/2 cup brown sugar, packed
3 tbsp half & half cream
1/3 cup chopped nuts
3/4 cup flaked coconut

Combine all ingredients. Spread evenly over warm cake. Broil until frosting becomes bubbly. (Approximately 2 minutes)

CHOCOLATE GLAZE

2 tbsp cocoa
1 tbsp oil
1 tbsp corn syrup
2 tbsp + 1 tsp water
1/2 tsp cinnamon (opt)
1 cup gluten-free icing sugar

In a small saucepan combine cocoa, oil, corn syrup, water and cinnamon. Stir over low heat until smooth. Gradually beat in sugar until smooth and shiny.

COCOA CREAM FROSTING

1 1/2 cup heavy cream, chilled
1/4 cup cocoa
3 tbsp brown sugar
1 tbsp gluten free icing sugar

Combine all ingredients in a medium sized bowl and beat until stiff. Frosting covers 2 - 8 inch cake layers.

OR Melt 1 square of semi-sweet chocolate. Remove from heat. In a large bowl, beat 3/4 cup heavy cream and 1 tbsp gluten-free icing sugar until stiff peaks form. Gradually beat in melted chocolate.

QUICK CHOCOLATE ICING

1 cup sugar

1/4 cup cocoa

1 tsp vanilla

1/4 cup evaporated milk

1/4 cup margarine

Put all ingredients in saucepan and heat on medium heat until mixture comes to a boil, stirring constantly. Boil 30 seconds and remove from heat without stirring. Cool until lukewarm. Add vanilla and beat until creamy enough to spread.

BAKERY SHOP ICING

1/2 cup margarine

2 tsp vanilla

6 tbsp shortening (Crisco)

1 tbsp cornstarch

1 cup white sugar

1/2 cup warm milk

Cream margarine, shortening, sugar, and vanilla in large bowl. Stir cornstarch into milk and then add to sugar mixture. Beat with electric mixer 5 - 7 minutes until very well blended.

1. Chocolate - add 1 square unsweetened chocolate (1 oz) and 1 tbsp cocoa to the mixture.
2. Various food colorings work well.

PASTRY I

1/2 cup creamed cottage cheese
1 egg
3/4 cup white rice flour
1/4 cup tapioca starch
1/4 cup cornstarch
1/4 cup potato starch
2 tbsp soya flour
1/2 tsp xanthan gum
3/4 tsp salt
1/2 cup lard (cold)

In a mixing bowl sift all the dry ingredients. In a blender combine the cottage cheese and egg until smooth. Set aside. Cut the hard lard into the dry ingredients until the size of split peas. Add the cottage cheese mix. Blend well with a fork. Knead lightly into a smooth dough. Chill. Roll out between 2 sheets of plastic wrap. Use as desired for pies or tarts.

For fruit pies bake at 425 F for 15 minutes, then reduce temperature to 350 F and bake another 30 - 50 minutes depending on filling and size of pie.

For baked shells, prick crust all over with fork and bake at 425 F about 10 - 15 minutes. Cool before filling with a cooked filling.

PASTRY II

1 cup + 2 tbsp brown rice flour
1 cup potato starch
1 tsp salt
1/2 cup lard (cold)
2 eggs, beaten

Sift dry ingredients into a mixing bowl. Cut in cold lard until size of split peas. Add beaten eggs and stir with a fork until well mixed (If the flour is especially dry 1 tbsp of ice water may have to be added). Knead lightly. Chill. Roll out pastry between two sheets of plastic wrap. Use as desired. Cool after baking before cutting.

Note: Pastry does not toughen when kneaded because there is no gluten. However do not overhandle as your warm hands will melt the lard and it will not be as tender and flaky.

RAISIN SOUR CREAM TARTS

1/2 cup brown sugar
1/2 tsp salt
1 tbsp cornstarch
1 egg
1 tsp vanilla
1/2 cup sour cream
1/2 cup raisins

1 dozen 2 inch tart shells - unbaked

Mix sugar, salt, and cornstarch together; then add rest of ingredients. Fill tart shells and bake at 400 F for approximately 15 - 20 minutes.

PUMPKIN TARTS

1/4 cup brown sugar
1/8 tsp salt
1/4 tsp cinnamon
1/8 tsp nutmeg
1/8 tsp cloves
2 eggs, beaten
3/4 cup canned pumpkin
1 tsp vanilla
1/2 cup whipped cream
1/2 cup finely chopped pecans
24 - 2 inch baked tart shells using Pastry I

In a pyrex bowl combine brown sugar, salt, and spices. Stir in eggs and pumpkin. Cook at medium in microwave for about 2 minutes until thickened. Add vanilla. Cover and chill completely. Fold in whipped topping. Spoon into baked tart shells. Top with chopped pecans. Refrigerate.

APRICOT FOLDOVERS

1/4 cup orange juice
4 tbsp sugar
1 cup dried apricots, finely chopped

Preheat oven to 350 F. In a small saucepan, mix above ingredients. Simmer, covered for 10 minutes, remove cover and simmer 10 more minutes, stirring occasionally until most of the liquid is absorbed. Cool. Grease 2 cookie sheets. Using pastry #1 roll out as before into a 10- inch square. Cut in 2 inch squares. Place 1/2 tsp apricot filling in center of each square. Moisten edges and fold dough diagonally over filling and press firmly to seal. Place on cookie sheet. Repeat with remaining dough and filling. Bake at 350 for 12 - 15 minutes. Let cool on wire rack.

FRESH PEACH PIE

1 - 8 oz cream cheese
1/3 cup milk
1/4 cup sugar
1 egg
1/2 tsp almond flavoring
1 1/2 cups sliced peaches

2 cups crushed gluten- free cornflakes
1/4 cup melted margarine
Blend cornflakes and margarine together, then press into
pie plate. Bake at 350 F for 5 minutes. Beat first five
ingredients together well, then fold in peaches. Pour filling
into crust and bake at 350 F for 25 - 30 minutes. Do not
overbake. Cool and top with whipped cream.

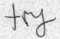

CHOCOLATE MALLOW PIE

1 baked meringue pie shell
(under Novelty Crust Section)
2/3 cup evaporated milk
1 square unsweetened chocolate
1 square semi-sweet chocolate
2 cups miniature or 32 large marshmallows
2 cups whipping cream

Combine milk, chocolate and marshmallows in top of
double boiler which has been placed over boiling water.
Heat the mixture until it is melted and smooth, stirring
constantly. Let cool to room temperature. Beat whipping
cream until stiff. Fold the cooled marshmallow mixture
into 1/4 of the whipped cream, then into remaining cream.
Spoon filling into a meringue crust. Chill 2-3 hours or
overnight.

GLUTEN FREE ANYTIME

NOVELTY CRUSTS

CRUMB PIE CRUST

1 cup brown rice flour
1/3 cup butter or margarine
4 tbsp brown sugar
1/2 cup chopped pecans or walnuts

Mix all ingredients together, spread in cake pan and bake for 15 minutes at 400 F. Remove from oven and stir with spoon. Use this for your favourite crumble recipe as a topping or immediately press 1 cup crumbs into sides of 9 inch pie plate. Cool and add your favourite pie filling and put remaining 3/4 cup mixture on top.

CRUMB CRUST

1 1/2 cups crumbs (using gluten-free cornflakes, rice krispies or cookie crumbs. Gingersnaps or gingerbread cookies are especially good)
1 tsp rice flour
2 tbsp sugar
1/4 cup melted butter or margarine

Mix all ingredients together and press firmly into a 9 inch buttered pie pan making an even layer.

SHAPING A CRUMB CRUST

To make a successful crumb crust you should have 2 pie plates each an inch different in size. After spreading the crumb mixture evenly over the bottom of a 9 inch plate, press an 8 inch pie plate firmly into the crumbs to distribute them evenly. Then press the inner plate firmly against the sides of the outer plate, all around, to push crumbs up the sides and into the rim. With your fingers,press crumbs firmly on the top of the rim to form an even edge all around. Remove inner pie plate.

MERINGUE CRUST

4 egg whites
1/4 tsp salt
1 tsp vinegar
1 cup granulated sugar

Preheat oven to 275 F. Grease and flour a 9 inch pie pan. Beat egg whites until frothy, add salt and vinegar. Continue beating until stiff. Gradually add 1 cup sugar, 2 tbsp at a time, beating thoroughly after each addition. Continue beating until all sugar is dissolved and mixture is very stiff and glossy. Spread in well greased and floured (with white rice flour) 9 inch pie pan, spreading some meringue up the sides of the pan. Bake in a slow oven 275 F for 1 1/2 hours. Cool. A lemon pie filling may be used to fill the shell. Cover with whipped cream.

JELLY ROLL

4 eggs
3/4 cup sugar
1 tsp vanilla

1/4 cup white rice flour
1/2 cup potato starch
1/4 tsp salt
1 1/2 tsp baking powder

Preheat oven to 375 F. Line a 15 1/2 x 10 1/2 baking sheet with waxed paper. Grease and lightly dust with potato starch.

Beat eggs in a deep bowl until fluffy and creamy. Add sugar gradually, beating after each addition. Add vanilla. Sift together flour, starch, baking powder, and salt. Sift dry ingredients gradually over egg mixture and fold in. Pour into prepared pan. Bake for 15 - 20 minutes. Meanwhile sift gluten-free icing sugar onto a clean kitchen towel over a 15 x 10 inch area. Turn out the cake onto the towel.

Remove waxed paper carefully and roll cake quickly with the towel. Allow to cool 15 minutes. Unroll and spread with jelly, jam, whipped cream or lemon filling 1/2 inch from edges. Roll again and cover with towel. Let cool. The roll may be sprinkled with gluten free icing sugar.

FILLINGS FOR JELLY ROLLS

CHOCOLATE FILLING
1 pkg dessert topping or 1 cup whipped cream
1 tbsp cocoa (sifted)
1 tsp peppermint flavor

MOCHA FILLING
1 pkg dessert topping or 1 cup whipped cream
1 tsp instant coffee
1 tbsp cocoa (sifted)

FRUIT FILLING
1 pkg dessert topping or whipped cream
Pureed fruit or baby fruit to taste

CREAM PUFFS

1 cup water (boiling)
1/2 cup butter or margarine
pinch salt
1/2 cup white rice flour
1/2 cup cornstarch
4 eggs
1 tsp sugar (optional)

Set oven to 425 F. Grease baking sheets. Measure butter, boiling water, salt and sugar if used, into a saucepan. Stir. Heat until butter melts and water comes to a full rolling boil. Sift flours together and add all at once, beating vigorously until mixture forms a ball - about one minute. Remove from heat; cool slightly. Add eggs one at a time, and beat until paste is smooth and shiny. Drop by spoonsful onto a greased baking sheet about 1 1/2 inch apart. Bake at 425 F for 15 minutes, and then reduce heat to 350 F for 20 minutes or until golden. Cut a slit in the side of each puff to allow steam to escape.

Return cream puffs to oven for 15 minutes longer . Turn off oven. Cool puffs on wire rack. Slice off top and fill with cream filling, whipped cream, or a filling of your choice. Replace top.

<u>FILLINGS</u>

1. Use prepared pudding mix using 1/2 cup less milk. Slice off top of each puff shell and spoon in pudding. Cover with top. Dust with gluten free icing sugar.

2. Whip 1 cup whipping cream or 1 pkg whipped topping mix. Whipped cream or topping mix can be flavored with 2 tsp cocoa and 1 tsp almond or peppermint flavoring beaten in when cream starts to thicken.

3. Make your own vanilla custard cream filling using cornstarch to thicken the filling. Use half as much cornstarch as flour that is called for in the recipe.

4. Fruit Mallow Filling - Combine 1 1/2 cups miniature marshmallows, 2 tbsp sugar and 3/4 cup sour cream. Chill, covered for 2 hours. Fold finely chopped fruit into chilled sour cream mixture.

ECLAIRS

The basic cream puff recipe can be shaped into eclairs, long finger length strips. A pastry bag and large tip can be used to shape the eclairs onto greased baking sheets. Bake at 400 F for 40 minutes. Turn off oven. Slit the end of eclairs to let steam escape and return to oven for 10 minutes. Remove from baking sheet to wire rack. Cool completely and fill with cream or other favourite filling by making a small hole in the end of each eclair. A decorating bag and a large tube works well to fill eclairs. Tops may be glazed with chocolate. Melt 2 squares of semi-sweet chocolate with 1 tbsp butter (or use chocolate chips) or the Chocolate Glaze recipe in the Cake - Frosting Section.

CREAM FILLING

2 cups milk
1/4 cup sugar
2 tbsp cornstarch
1/4 tsp salt
3 egg yolks
1 tsp vanilla
1 tbsp butter

Mix sugar, cornstarch and salt together. Gradually add
milk mixing well to a smooth mixture. Cook in microwave
on HI for 3 minutes then MOD for about 2 more minutes
stirring several times until thickened. (Mixture can be
cooked in a double boiler until thickened). Beat egg yolks
slightly, blend a bit of the hot mixture with the yolks,
stirring constantly, then add all to the milk - cornstarch
mixture. Cook on MOD for 1 minute (about 3 - 4 minutes
over the simmering water). Beat in the vanilla and butter.
Cool, fill cake or pour into pie shell. The pie can be topped
with meringue made from the egg whites.

<u>LEMON FILLING</u>

4 tbsp cornstarch
1/4 tsp salt
3/4 cup granulated sugar
2 cups boiling water
1 tbsp grated lemon rind
4 tbsp lemon juice
2 egg yolks, slightly beaten
1/4 cup butter

Add lemon rind to boiling water. Mix cornstarch, salt, and sugar together. Slowly add the boiling water to mix, stirring constantly. Microwave (or cook in saucepan MOD heat) on HI for 3 minutes approximately stirring every 30 seconds until thickened. Add a little of the hot mixture to the egg yolks, mix well, and return the egg yolk mixture to the entire amount of hot mixture stirring constantly. Cook on MOD for 1 minute in microwave or until well cooked in the saucepan on the stove. Remove from heat and beat in lemon juice and butter until well blended. Cool. This can be used as a filling for a layer cake or pie. For a lemon cream (fluffy) filling; fold in 1/2 cup whipped cream when lemon filling is cold.

GLUTEN FREE ANYTIME

RICE DESSERT

1 pkg orange jelly powder
1 cup cooked rice
1 cup dream whip, prepared
1 cup chopped pecans (opt)
1 cup crushed pineapple, drained
1 cup small marshmallows

Dissolve jelly powder in 1 cup hot water. Use 1 cup of pineapple juice, or juices and water to make up the other cup of liquid. When jelly is nearly set, whip and add other ingredients. Refrigerate for several hours before serving.

CREAMY APPLE CHEESE BAKE

1 cup "Gluten Free Anytime" Mix
1 tbsp sugar
pinch salt
1/4 cup cold margarine
1 egg yolk, slightly beaten
1 tsp water

To make crust, sift dry ingredients together into a bowl.
Cut in cold margarine. Combine the egg yolk with 1 tsp
water and blend into crumb mixture. Press on bottom and
sides of an 8 x 8 x 2 inch pan.

2 1/2 cups canned sliced apples, drained
1/3 cup sugar
1 tsp lemon juice
1/4 tsp cinnamon
1/4 tsp nutmeg

Combine and turn into crust. Bake at 425 F for 10 minutes.

1/2 cup sugar
pinch salt
2 slightly beaten eggs
8 oz cream cheese
1/2 cup whipping cream
1 tsp vanilla

Mix together sugar, salt, and blend into the beaten eggs and
cream cheese. Mix in the cream and vanilla. Pour over
apples. Bake at 350 F for 30 minutes or until set. Chill
thoroughly. Makes 8 - 9 servings.

GLUTEN FREE ANYTIME

<u>APPLE CRISP</u>

4 cups sliced pared cored apples
2/3 cup brown sugar
1/2 cup sifted rice flour
1/2 cup corn germ
3/4 tsp cinnamon
3/4 tsp nutmeg
1/3 cup soft butter

Place apples in a greased 8 inch square pan. Blend remaining ingredients until crumbly, spread over apples. Bake at 375 F for 30 - 35 minutes. Serve with ice cream or whipped cream. Makes 6 servings.

APPLE RAISIN CRISP

1/3 cup "Gluten Free Anytime" Mix
1 cup corn germ
1/3 cup brown sugar, packed
1/2 cup margarine, melted
1/8 tsp salt
4 cups sliced apples (4 - 5 medium)
1/2 cup raisins
1/2 cup sugar
2 tbsp water
2 tsp lemon juice
1/2 tsp cinnamon

Preheat oven to 375 F. Grease an 8 inch square pan or 1 1/2 quart casserole dish. Sift mix into bowl. Add corn germ and brown sugar. Stir until well blended. Add melted margarine and blend well with a fork. Arrange apples and raisins in a greased pan. Sprinkle with sugar, water, lemon juice, and cinnamon. Sprinkle crisp topping over the fruit. Bake until fruit is tender, about 35 minutes. Serve warm or cold with whipped cream if desired.

RHUBARB CRISP

Use the crisp topping as above. Prepare fruit mixture using 4 cups fresh cut up rhubarb or well drained frozen rhubarb. Sprinkle 3/4 cup sugar and 1/2 tsp cinnamon over the fruit. Prepare and bake as for Apple Raisin Crisp.

BLUEBERRY COBBLER

4 cups blueberries
2 tbsps cornstarch
2 tbsp lemon juice
1/2 tsp cinnamon, optional
1/2 cup granulated sugar

1 3/4 cups "Gluten Free Anytime " Mix
4 tsp baking powder
1/4 tsp salt
1/2 cup chilled margarine
1 egg
1/2 cup milk

Preheat oven to 375 F.
Mix thoroughly the blueberries, cornstarch, lemon juice,
1/4 cup sugar, and cinnamon if used, and put into a 10 inch
deep round dish. Set aside. Measure mix, 1/4 cup sugar,
baking powder, and salt into a medium sized mixing bowl.
Cut in margarine until crumbly. Make a well in center. In a
separate bowl beat egg and milk together and pour into
well. Stir just until mixed. Drop spoonsful of batter over
entire surface of blueberries. Bake 45 minutes or until
cobbler is golden. Serve warm or cold with whipped
cream.

<u>GINGERBREAD (OLD TIME)</u>

1/3 cup shortening
1/2 cup granulated sugar
2 eggs, beaten
1/2 cup light molasses

1 cup white rice flour
1/4 cup corn flour
1/2 cup potato starch
1 tsp cinnamon
1 tsp ginger
1 tsp unflavored gelatin
1 1/2 tsp baking powder
1 tsp baking soda
1/4 cup buttermilk

Preheat oven to 350 F. Grease and flour (gluten-free) an 8 x 8 inch pan. Cream shortening and sugar. Add molasses, blending well. Then add eggs and mix well. Sift flours, starch, salt, baking powder, and unflavored gelatin. Dissolve baking soda in buttermilk; add alternately with flour mixture to molasses mixture. Pour into prepared pan. Bake for 45 minutes or until toothpick comes out clean. Cool on rack before cutting. Serve with whipped cream or lemon sauce.

LEMON SAUCE

1/2 cup granulated sugar
1 1/2 tbsp cornstarch
1 1/2 tsp grated lemon rind
1 cup hot water
2 1/2 tbsp lemon juice
1 tbsp butter

Combine sugar, lemon rind, and cornstarch in a small saucepan. Stir in hot water. Cook over medium heat until thickened and clear, stirring constantly. Remove from heat and add lemon juice and butter. Serve hot or cold. Makes about 1 cup.

RAISIN PUDDING

1/2 cup brown sugar
1/2 tsp salt
1 cup rice flour
1 cup raisins
2 tsp baking powder
1/2 cup milk

Mix the above in an oven proof bowl. Mix the following ingredients and pour over the above.
1 1/2 cups brown sugar
1 1/2 cups boiling water

1 1/2 tbsp butter
1 tsp nutmeg or cinnamon

Bake at 350 F for 3/4 hour. Insert toothpick in the center of pudding - when it comes out clean the pudding is done. This is very sweet and small portions are adequate. This will serve 4.

RICE PUDDING

1/2 cup rice
1 cup water
3 cups milk
1 tsp grated orange peel
1/2 cup sugar
1/8 tsp salt
1 tbsp margarine or butter
2 egg yolks
1/2 cup light raisins
1 tsp vanilla extract

Put the rice and water in a heavy saucepan. Bring to a boil and cover; boil 5 minutes stirring occasionally. Stir in the milk, sugar, orange peel, salt and butter. Cook, covered over boiling water 45 minutes, or until rice is tender. Stir occasionally. Beat the egg yolks slightly; gradually add a little of the hot mixture to the yolks while stirring constantly. Add yolk mixture to the hot mixture, with the raisins and vanilla. Stir to blend, cover and chill thoroughly. Top with cream and a sprinkle of cinnamon.

BROWNIE PUDDING

1/2 cup white rice flour
1/2 cup potato starch
1/2 cup sugar
2 tbsp cocoa
2 tsp baking powder
1/2 tsp salt
1/4 cup chopped nuts
1/2 cup milk
2 tbsp melted margarine
1 tsp vanilla
1/2 cup brown sugar, packed
1/4 cup cocoa
1 1/2 cups hot water

Preheat oven to 350 F. Grease a 8 x 8 x 2 inch pan.
Sift flour and starch together, then sift the flour, starch,
sugar, baking powder, salt, and 2 tbsp cocoa together into a
mixing bowl. Stir in nuts. Add milk, vanilla, and melted
margarine. Mix well. Pour into prepared pan. Combine
brown sugar and 1/4 cup cocoa. Sprinkle evenly over
batter. Pour hot water carefully over entire batter. Do not
stir. Bake for 40 - 45 minutes. Serve warm with ice cream
or whipped cream. Makes 6 servings.

CAKE TOP PUDDING
(a light cake on top with a sauce below)

1/4 cup sifted "Gluten Free Anytime" Mix
3/4 cup granulated sugar
1/4 tsp salt
1 tbsp grated orange peel
1/2 cup orange juice
2 eggs, separated
3/4 cup milk

Preheat oven to 350 F. Grease a 1 quart baking dish. Sift flour, sugar, and salt together. Blend in orange peel, egg yolks, orange juice, and milk. Beat egg whites until stiff but not dry. Fold in the orange mixture gently. Pour into prepared pan, set pan in another pan which contains 1 inch depth of hot water. Bake 45 - 50 minutes. Makes 6 servings.

LEMON CAKE PUDDING

As above but substitute the 1 tbsp orange rind for 1 1/2 tsp lemon rind and the 1/2 cup orange juice for 1/4 cup lemon juice and extra 1/4 cup milk.

Cheese Cake.

CHERRY DELIGHT

1 1/2 cups crushed gluten free cornflakes
1/4 cup melted margarine

8 oz cream cheese
1/2 cup sugar
1 tsp vanilla
1 pkg Dream Whip
1/2 cup milk
1 can Cherry or Blueberry pie filling

Add margarine to cornflakes, mix well and press into pie plate. Bake at 350 F for 5 minutes. Cream the cheese, adding sugar and vanilla, beating until fluffy. Add the Dream Whip and milk to the cheese mixture and whip until stiff. Then pour into the crust and refrigerate overnight. Top with pie filling before serving.

MALLOW CREAM WHIP

16 large or 2 cups miniature marshmallows
3/4 cup orange juice
1/2 cup whipping cream, whippped

In a saucepan (or in a pyrex bowl if using a microwave) over low heat melt marshmallows in the juice stirring constantly. Quickly chill to consistency of egg white. Beat until foamy, then fold in whipped cream. Pour into sherbet glasses. Refrigerate several hours.

FRUIT PIZZA
(a dessert that can be used with a variety of fruits)

Crust:
- 1/2 cup butter or good quality margarine
- 1/4 cup gluten-free icing sugar
- 1 cup "Gluten Free Anytime" Mix

Filling:
- 3 tbsp peach or apricot jam, melted
- 4 oz cream cheese
- 2 tsp grated orange rind
- 1/2 cup whipping cream
- 4 - 5 apples, peaches, pears(peeled, pitted, & sliced)

Glaze:
- 2 tbsp cornstarch
- 3 tbsp brown sugar
- 3/4 cup orange juice
- 1/2 cup apricot or peach jam
- whipped cream

Preheat oven to 350 F.

<u>Crust:</u> In a mixing bowl combine flour and icing sugar. Cut in butter until crumbly. The mixture should hold together when pressed together with fingers. Pat evenly onto a 10 inch pizza pan. Prick crust all over with a fork. Bake 15 - 20 minutes or until golden. Cool.

Filling: Brush the crust with melted jam to seal the crust. Beat together the cream cheese, orange rind and whipping cream until smooth. Spread over crust. Arrange fruit slices on top in a pleasing pattern.

Glaze: Mix cornstarch and brown sugar together in a saucepan (or in a 2 cup glass bowl if using a microwave). Add rest of ingredients and blend. Cook over medium heat stirring constantly until mixture bubbles and becomes thick and clear. Let cool slightly and spoon over fruit. (If using the microwave heat on Med High and cook for approximately 2 - 3 minutes stirring each minute during the cooking time). Garnish the pizza with whipped cream.

STRAWBERRY PIZZA

Substitute fresh sliced strawberries for other fruit and then use a plain or fruit glaze to cover fruit. (eg. MPK Glaze, Oetker which are gluten free)

GLUTEN FREE ANYTIME

A. CRISPY COATING SUGGESTIONS

Use any of the following:
1 cup rolled potato chips OR
1 cup taco chips OR
Cornmeal OR
Corngerm OR
Instant potato flakes plus parmesan cheese mixed together
season with salt and pepper
Always roll meat, fish, poultry in one of the following:
melted butter, evaporated milk, beaten eggs and then into
the crumbs, cornmeal etc.

B. COATING MIX FOR CHICKEN

1/2 cup "Gluten Free Anytime" Mix
1 tsp onion salt
1 tsp garlic salt
1/4 tsp salt
1 tsp dried parsley flakes
1 1/2 tsp thyme
1/2 tsp paprika
1/4 tsp pepper

Mix all together. Moisten chicken with water or evaporated
milk. Place mix in plastic bag and then add chicken one
piece at a time and shake to coat. Place on greased baking
sheet and bake at 400 F for about 40 minutes, turning once
during baking.

C. ITALIAN FLAVORED COATING MIX

1 cup "Gluten Free Anytime" Mix
1 tsp oregano
1/2 tsp basil
2 tbsp Parmesan cheese
Use as above.

RICE STUFFING

1/2 cup margarine
2 cups chopped celery
1 1/2 cup chopped onions
1/2 cup chopped mushrooms
2 tsp salt
1 tsp sage
1 tsp thyme
1/4 tsp pepper
6 cups cooked brown rice (cooked in chicken broth if possible)
2 eggs, beaten

Melt margarine in a large frying pan. Saute onions, celery, and mushrooms. Mix in spices and rice. Stir in beaten eggs and mix very thoroughly. Stuff turkey. (Makes about 10 cups of stuffing). The stuffing may also be cooked in a large greased casserole and bake at 350 F for about 1 hour.

RICE AND VEGETABLE STUFFING

1 cup grated carrots
1/2 cup chopped onion
1/2 cup chopped parsley
4 tbsp margarine or butter
3 cups chicken broth
1 cup regular uncooked rice
1/2 tsp salt
1/8 tsp pepper
1/2 tsp sage

Cook carrots, onions, and parsley in margarine or butter for 10 minutes. Add uncooked rice. Stir to mix well. Add broth, spices. Cook covered until rice is done about 20 minutes. The stuffing may also be baked in a greased, covered 1 1/2 quart casserole at 375 F for 20 - 25 minutes.

RICE PIZZA CRUST

1 1/2 cups cooked rice
2 eggs, beaten
2 tbsp finely chopped onion
1/2 cup grated mozzarella cheese

Mix and press mixture evenly with a spoon into a greased
10 or 12 inch pizza pan or form into a circle onto greased
baking pan. Bake at 450 F about 20 minutes or until lighty
browned. Remove from oven and prepare your favourite
pizza sauce and toppings. Bake about 10 minutes longer or
until cheese melts, if using fresh grated cheese.

POTATO CRUST

3 cups raw potatoes, peeled & grated
3 tbsp butter, melted

Toss butter and grated potatoes together and press into a 9
inch pie plate. Bake at 450 F for 15 minutes. Use as a crust
for any quiche filling.

PIZZA CRUST

1/2 cup potato starch
1/2 cup cornstarch
1 tbsp baking powder
1/2 tsp baking soda
1/4 tsp salt
1 cup milk
1/4 cup melted margarine
1 egg, beaten
1/2 cup instant mashed potato flakes

Preheat oven to 400 F. Grease well a 12 inch pizza pan. Mix together first five ingredients. Mix egg, milk, and margarine together and add all at once to dry ingredients. Mix well. Blend in potato flakes. Pour onto prepared pan spreading to edges of the pan. Bake for 15 minutes or until crust is golden brown. Remove from oven and add your tomato sauce, seasonings, and favorite toppings like bacon and mushroom, ham and pineapple, or just cheese. Return to hot oven until cheese is melted and bubbly.

BROWN RICE CRUST FOR QUICHE OR PIZZA

2 1/2 cups cooked brown rice (takes about 45 min. to cook)
1 egg, slightly beaten
1/2 cup grated Swiss cheese

Mix together and press into a 9 - 10 inch pie or quiche pan.

LASAGNA TIP

Use cooked rice or sliced zucchini in place of lasagna noodles and layer as usual.

ZUCCHINI QUICHE #1

6 slices bacon, cooked crisp and crumbled
(Save 2 tbsp fat)
1/2 cup chopped onions
2 cups coarsely grated zucchini
1 tsp salt
1/2 tsp oregano
1/2 tsp basil
1/8 tsp pepper
3 eggs, slightly beaten
1/2 cup evaporated milk (or half & half)

Cook onions and zucchini in the 2 tbsp bacon fat until just tender. Add oregano, basil, salt and pepper. Place crumbled bacon in rice crust, cover with the onions and zucchini. Mix the eggs and milk and pour over the vegetables. Bake at 375 F for 30 minutes. Cool a few minutes before cutting into wedges. Makes 6 servings.

ZUCCHINI QUICHE #2

4 eggs, slightly beaten
3 cups shredded zucchini
1/2 onion, finely chopped
1/2 cup cooking oil
1 cup grated marble cheese
7/8 cup brown rice flour
2 1/2 tsp baking powder
1 tsp salt
1 tbsp parsley, chopped
1/2 tsp each marjoram, oregano
dash cayenne
dash pepper
dash garlic powder

Grease a 9 x 13 inch pan. Mix altogether and put into prepared pan. Top with 1/2 cup grated parmesan cheese. Bake 40 minutes at 375 F.

BROCCOLI QUICHE

Instead of zucchini, in Zucchini Quiche #1 recipe use 1 cup fresh or frozen broccoli. Cook until crisp tender if using fresh broccoli or cook frozen broccoli as directed on the package. Drain broccoli well. Omit crumbled bacon and use 1/2 cup cooked or drained, canned chopped mushrooms instead.

QUICHE LORRAINE

6 slices bacon
1/2 cup chopped onions
2 cups shredded Swiss Cheese (8 oz)
4 eggs
2 cups milk
1/4 tsp ground nutmeg
1 tsp salt
1/8 tsp pepper

Use unbaked pie shell for a 9 inch pie pan or quiche pan.
Preheat oven to 425 F. Prick unbaked pie shell all over
with a fork. Bake in a hot oven (425 F) for 5 minutes. Cool
slightly on a wire rack. Increase oven temperature to 450 F.

Fry bacon until crisp, drain all but 1 tbsp fat. Crumble
bacon. Saute onion in bacon fat until cooked. Sprinkle
cheese evenly over the partly baked pie shell. Add bacon
and onion. Beat eggs slightly, slowly beat in milk and
seasonings, then pour into pastry shell. Bake at 450 F for
15 minutes. Lower oven temperature to 350 F for 15
minutes or until center is almost set by inserting a knife
into filling and it should come out almost clean. Let stand
for 15 minutes when the filling will set completely.
  *If not using pastry, grease pie pan well and continue as if
a pastry shell was used. Set oven to 450 F, fry bacon, saute
onion and so on.*

CHICKEN STOCK FOR SOUP

6 cups water
stewing hen, parts of chicken
1/2 gingerroot
1 tbsp sugar
1 1/2 tsp salt
Boil together until chicken is tender.

BEEF STOCK FOR SOUPS
(Use beef shank, round bone roast or short ribs)

8 - 10 cups water
celery leaves
fresh parsley
1 onion, chopped coarsely
1 carrot, sliced
2 bay leaves
8 - 10 peppercorns
2 whole cloves
1 1/2 tsp salt (or to taste)

Bring water and meat to a slow boil, skim, and simmer for
1 hour. Add greens, vegetables and spices. Simmer for
another hour or more. Remove meat and use as desired.
Strain the stock.

Serving Ideas for Beef Broth

1. Bring 2 cups of beef stock to a boil, then add leftover cooked rice or cooked pastas.

2. Bring 2 cups of stock to a boil, then add 3 tbsp cream of rice. Cook for 3 minutes. Serve hot.

3. Beat 2 eggs, 1 tbsp cornstarch, and 1 tbsp water together. Add 1/4 tsp nutmeg. Add to 4 cups boiling stock. Take off heat and serve.

4. Drop spoonsful of dumplings into 4 cups boiling stock. Cover pot and simmer for 12 - 15 minutes. No peeking!

5. Any amount or kind of diced vegetables may be added to stock.

CREAM SOUPS
(A thin white sauce is the basis for cream soups)

White Cream Sauce:
1/4 cup margarine or butter
1 cup milk
4 tbsp brown or white rice flour (or 2 tbsp cornstarch)
1/4 tsp salt
fresh ground pepper

Melt butter and add the flour (cornstarch is mixed with the cold milk and then poured into the melted butter). Add milk, stir over medium heat until thickened. Add seasonings.

Cream Of Potato Soup

2 cups white sauce + 1/2 cup potato water or
additional milk
1 cup cooked mashed or diced potatoes
1/8 tsp onion salt
1/2 tsp dried parsley
1/2 tsp celery salt

Combine mashed potato and potato water/milk. Add to white sauce which has had the seasonings added. Heat and serve.

Cream of Tomato Soup

2 cups canned tomatoes
1/2 tsp sugar
2 tbsp fat
2 cups milk
1 slice onion or 1/4 tsp onion salt
1 1/2 tbsp cornstarch
1 tsp salt
few grains pepper

Cook tomatoes with onion, sugar, and seasonings. Put through a sieve to remove seeds. Make a thin tomato sauce using sieved tomatoes as liquid instead of milk in the white sauce recipe. Just before serving add sauce to cold milk stirring it in gradually. Heat and serve at once. Do not boil as mixture will curdle.

Cream of Vegetable Soup

2 cups white sauce
1/2 cup milk
1 cup chopped raw vegetables
1 cup water or stock
1/2 tsp celery salt
1/4 tsp onion salt

Cook vegetables in water. Make white sauce. Add vegetables and seasonings. Heat and serve.

try

HAMBURGER SOUP #1

1 tbsp butter
2 lbs hamburger
2 cups diced potatoes
1 cup corn
2 cups shredded cabbage
1 cup diced celery
1 cup diced carrots
2 cups diced onions
2 quarts hot water
2 cups tomatoes
1/4 cup rice
1 1/2 tsp salt

Melt butter, add meat and brown. Add vegetables and water. Bring back to a boil, add rice and salt. Simmer 1 - 1 1/2 hours (or make it in a slow cooker, let cook all day). Freezes well.

HAMBURGER SOUP #2

1 lb ground beef
1 tsp each pepper and salt
1 quart of water
1 medium onion, chopped
1 tbsp cornstarch
1/4 - 1/2 cup cream
1 egg
5 medium potatoes, cooked
1 tbsp pickling spices
1/4 cup each vinegar & water

Mix beef, egg, salt and pepper and shape into small meat
balls. Bring 1 quart water to a boil in large saucepan. Add
pickling spices and onion, then simmer for 5 minutes. Add
meat balls to simmering mixture and continue cooking for
10 - 15 minutes until meat balls are cooked. Mix cornstarch
and 1/4 cup water until smooth and add to simmering
mixture and cook another 5 minutes. Remove from heat,
then add cream (depending on how rich you desire the
soup) and serve at once over boiled potatoes in soup bowls.

AUTUMN SOUP

1 lb ground beef
1 cup diced potatoes
1 tsp meat extract
1 cup chopped onions
2 tsp salt
1 bay leaf
1 cup diced celery
1/2 tsp pepper
pinch of basil
6 whole fresh tomatoes or 1 can tomatoes

Brown meat slowly in hot fat in heavy skillet. Add onions and cook about 5 minutes. Loosen meat from bottom of kettle. Add remaining ingredients except tomatoes. Bring to boil, cover, and simmer 20 minutes. Add tomatoes, simmer 10 minutes more. Nutritious for dieters.

CABBAGE BEAN SOUP

1/4 cup chopped onion
3 medium potatoes, peeled & diced
1 lb cabbage (approximately 6 cups)
1 clove garlic
1/2 tsp poultry seasoning
1 can beans & pork with tomato sauce
1 large rib celery, thinly sliced
2 tbsp oil
3 cups chicken broth
1 bay leaf
1/2 tsp each of salt and pepper

Saute onion, celery, potatoes in oil. Stir in cabbage, cover and cook over moderate heat stirring occasionally for 10 minutes until cabbage cooks down. Add remaining ingredients except beans. Cover and simmer 20 minutes or until potatoes and cabbage are tender, stirring occasionally. Stir in beans. Cook 10 minutes longer for beans to heat.

DUMPLINGS

1/2 cup white rice flour
1/4 cup soya flour
1/4 cup potato starch
1/4 tsp xanthan gum
1/2 tsp salt
2 1/2 tsp baking powder
1/2 cup milk
2 tbsp melted margarine, chicken or beef fat

<u>Beef Broth</u> - season with 1/4 tsp pepper, 1/4 tsp dried
parsley

<u>Chicken broth</u> - season with 1/4 tsp thyme &
1/4 tsp poultry seasoning

Boil soup broth. Sift together flours, starch, gum, salt,
baking powder, and seasonings into medium sized bowl.
Stir in melted fat and milk. Dip tablespoon into boiling
broth, then into dough and drop spoonful of dough into
gently boiling broth. When all dough is used, cover broth
and steam without lifting cover for 12 - 15 minutes. Serve
hot in the soup broth.

<u>POPOVERS</u>

1/2 cup white rice flour
1/2 cup cornstarch or potato starch
1/2 tsp salt
2 eggs
1 cup milk
2 tsp melted shortening

Heat oven to 425 F. Grease muffin tins or custard cups
very well. Sift together the rice flour and corn/potato
starch. Beat eggs slightly in a bowl. Add the rest of the
ingredients and beat with mixer until smooth. Fill muffin
tins 1/3 to 1/2 full. Bake for 15 minutes at 450 F, reduce
heat to 350 F for another 25 - 30 minutes or until crisp to
the touch. Prick each popover with a skewer or fork to let
steam escape. Turn off oven and let popovers remain in
oven 10 minutes longer. If they are not crisp, popovers will
collapse. (Makes 10 popovers)

Popovers may be served with jam or jelly, as a container
for creamed foods (creamed chicken, fish, vegetables)
when the top is cut and the creamed mixture is spooned
inside, and as a substitute for Yorkshire pudding. Recipe
can be halved to make 5 - 6 popovers.

YORKSHIRE PUDDING

1/2 cup sifted "Gluten Free Anytime" Mix
1/2 tsp salt
3/4 cup milk
2 eggs, slightly beaten
2 tbsp melted beef fat or drippings or oil

Mix flour and salt together then place in blender and add milk a little at a time, blending until smooth. Add eggs and beat until bubbly about 2 - 3 minutes. Cover loosely and let stand in a cool place about 30 minutes. (Do not refrigerate). Preheat oven to 450 F. Beat batter again 1 - 2 minutes until bubbly. Pour 1/2 tsp fat into each of 10 muffin pan cups and heat in oven 1 - 2 minutes until pan is very hot. Spoon or pour 3 tbsp of batter into each muffin cup (or fill to 1/2) and bake 12 minutes. Reduce heat to 400 F and bake about 10 minutes longer until well browned puffy and crisp. Arrange around a beef roast and serve at once.

GLUTEN FREE ANYTIME

GLUTEN FREE ANYTIME

I wish to order: _____ Cookbooks @ 16.95 (less than 10)
Gluten Free Anytime _____ Cookbooks @ 12.95 (11 to 24)
_____ Cookbooks @ 11.95 (over 25)
Book fees enclosed: _____ **for Book #1 (Beige Book)**
Postage _____ ($3.00 per individual book)
Total _____ (Bulk orders- postage payable)
(payable to *Gluten Free Anytime)* (upon receipt of books)

Name: _____
Address: _____
City: _____
Postal Code: _____

MAIL TO :

Gluten Free Anytime
583 Cottonwood Ave.
* Prices July 1997 **Sherwood Park, Alberta**
subject to change* **T8A 1Y5**

I wish to order: _____ Cookbooks @ 16.95 (less than 10)
Gluten Free Anytime _____ Cookbooks @ 12.95 (11 to 24)
Special _____ Cookbooks @ 11.95 (over 25)
Book fees enclosed: _____ **For Cookbook #2 (Pink Book)**
Postage _____ ($3.00 per individual book)
Total _____ (Bulk orders- postage payable)
(payable to *Gluten Free Anytime)* (upon receipt of books)

Name: _____
Address: _____
City: _____
Postal Code: _____

MAIL TO:

Gluten Free Anytime
* Prices July 1997 **583 Cottonwood Ave.**
subject to change* **Sherwood Park, Alberta**
T8A 1Y5

GLUTEN FREE ANYTIME